OXFORD MEDICAL PUBLICATIONS

Radiology: a casebook for MRCP

D1757767

Radiology: a casebook for MRCP

CJ Harvey

Specialist Registrar in Radiology, The University College London Hospitals Trust, London UK

HRS Roberts

Senior Registrar in Radiology, The University College London Hospitals Trust, London UK

PJ Shaw

Consultant Radiologist, Dept of Imaging, The University College London Hospitals Trust, London UK

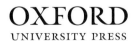

OXFORD

UNIVERSITY PRESS

OXFORD

UNIVERSITY PRESS

Great Clarendon Street, Oxford OX2 6DP

Oxford New York

Athens Auckland Bangkok Bogota Buenos Aires Calcutta
Cape Town Chennai Dar es Salaam Delhi Florence Hong Kong Istanbul
Karachi Kuala Lumpur Madrid Melbourne Mexico City Mumbai
Nairobi Paris São Paolo Singapore Taipei Tokyo Toronto Warsaw

and associated companies in
Berlin Ibadan

Oxford is a trade mark of Oxford University Press

Published in the United States
by Oxford University Press, Inc., New York

A catalogue record for this book is available from the British Library

Library of Congress Cataloging in Publication Data

Harvey, C. J. (Chris J.)
Radiology: a casebook for MRCP / C. J. Harvey, H. R. S. Roberts, P. J. Shaw.
(Oxford medical publications)
1. Radiography, Medical—Examinations, questions, etc.
I. Roberts, H. R. S. (Hugh R. S.)   II. Shaw, P. J. (Penny J.)
III. Title.   IV. Series.
[DNLM: 1. Diagnostic Imaging examination questions.   WN 18.2
H341r   1999]
RC78.15.H37   1999   616.07'54'076—dc21   98–49160
ISBN 0 19 262902 6 (Pbk)

Typeset by EXPO Holdings, Malaysia

Printed in Great Britain by
The Bath Press, Avon

We dedicate this book to our families who supported us during the preparation of this book.

C.H., H.R., P.S.

Foreword

by Professor Peter Dawson

In the one hundred years since the discovery of X-rays the specialty of radiology has revolutionized medical practice. The importance of this specialty is reflected by the fact that almost every patient seeking medical attention requires radiological imaging in one form or another. Consequently the MRCP candidate and medical student will be expected to be competent in the radiological interpretation of a wide range of commonly encountered and emergency conditions. With the changes in medical training and ever increasing knowledge base required of the prospective MRCP candidate, an updated radiological text specifically aimed at the needs of the examinee is particularly welcome.

The purpose of this book is to provide a set of images for the physician in training to improve competence in radiological interpretation and to guide the choice of appropriate imaging. Its success in these aims must therefore be judged by the choice and quality of the chosen images. *Radiology: a casebook for the MRCP* combines excellent quality images, detailed descriptions, and differentials, with up-to-date imaging strategies. Images of conditions frequently seen in the MRCP examination are, of course, well represented and are supplemented by a range of 'bread and butter' images covering a wide spectrum of clinical medicine. On these measures it succeeds admirably, as would be expected from these authors: an experienced teaching hospital consultant and two senior registrars who are well equipped for the task. Computed tomography, ultrasound, magnetic resonance imaging, and nuclear medicine are all represented. This book would benefit not only MRCP candidates and more experienced clinicians wishing to improve their radiological skills, but also trainees in radiology.

Preface

Diagnostic radiology plays a vital role in patient management and it is therefore essential that all clinicians are able to recognize the radiological appearances of a wide spectrum of medical conditions, both in their long-term clinical practice and in the short term to satisfy their examiners. Both graduate and postgraduate examinations, especially the written section of the MRCP (part II), contain a substantial amount of radiographic material. As well as the traditional imaging modalities, newer techniques such as interventional radiology, computed tomography (including helical CT), magnetic resonance imaging (MRI), nuclear medicine, and ultrasound form an increasing proportion of the cases. It is for this reason that a self assessment slide question/answer book illustrating these modalities, along with the more traditional techniques, is warranted. The cases discussed in this book cover the majority of the material likely to be encountered in the MRCP and final medical examinations. For a particular condition, examples of other modalities are given to show how the newer techniques contribute to the diagnostic process. In each case, the radiographic appearances are explained and the radiological investigation of the condition discussed. The book covers a wide spectrum of medical specialties in a systematic approach whilst retaining an examination paper 'feel'.

This book is aimed at not only those preparing for examinations, but also clinicians wishing to strengthen their radiological knowledge.

London   C.J.H.
1998   H.R.S.R.
                                                                                                        P.J.S.

Acknowledgements

The authors would like to thank Dr David Rickards, Dr Margaret Hall-Craggs, Dr Kate Walmsley, Dr Peter Renton, Dr Michael Kellett, Dr Caroline Parks, Dr Maurice Raphael, and Dr S. Garcinovic of the Middlesex and University College Hospitals, London, and Dr Clive Bartram of St Mark's Hospital, Harrow who generously donated radiographs, read manuscripts, and gave encouragement during the preparation of this book. We would also like to thank Helen Patterson and colleagues in the Department of Medical Photography, Middlesex Hospital for the excellent quality of the prints.

Contents

Abbreviations

ACTH	adrenocorticotrophic hormone
AXR	abdominal radiograph
CT	computed tomography
CXR	chest radiograph
ERCP	endoscopic retrograde cholangiopancreatography
ESR	erythrocyte sedimentation rate
FSH	follicle stimulating hormone
GH	growth hormone
IVU	intravenous urogram
LH	luteinizing hormone
MRI	magnetic resonance imaging
Nuc Med	nuclear medicine
SXR	skull radiograph
TSH	thyroid-stimulating hormone
US	ultrasound

NEUROLOGY

Question 1

This 14-year-old boy presented with a first grand mal fit. History revealed that he had learning difficulties at school. It was also noted that he had a long-standing facial rash.

What does this investigation show and what is the diagnosis?

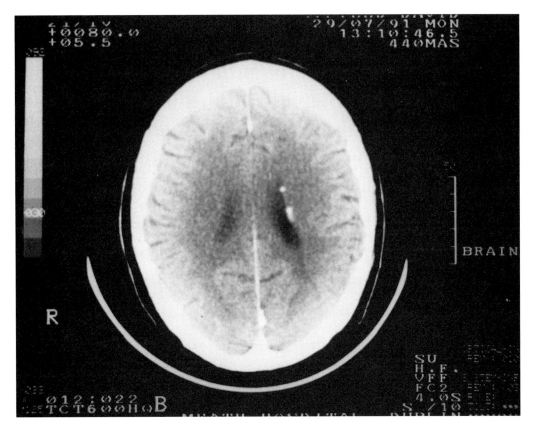

Fig. 1

Answer 1: Tuberous sclerosis

Findings: The axial unenhanced computed tomography (CT) scan taken at the level of the lateral ventricles shows characteristic periventricular calcified tubers. The differential for this appearance is intrauterine cytomegalovirus/toxoplasma infection but in these conditions smaller calcific lesions, cerebral atrophy, and microcephaly would also be present. The lateral skull radiograph (Fig. 1a) shows scattered areas of intracranial calcification (arrows) for which there is a long differential diagnosis.

Tuberous sclerosis is one of the hereditary phakomatoses (autosomal dominant) in which clinical manifestations are due to hamartomatous malformations of the brain, skin, heart, lung, and kidneys.

Involvement of the central nervous system is typically by periventricular tubers which commonly calcify and are classically described as having the appearance of candle wax dripping into the lateral ventricles. They may also occur in the cortical white matter or less commonly in the cerebellum. Tubers may transform into gliomas and a common site of occurrence is the foramen of Monro resulting in hydrocephalus. CT is the imaging modality of choice for diagnosing tuberous sclerosis as it is more sensitive than plain skull radiography for detecting intracranial calcification and a high proportion of patients show calcified tubers in early childhood. Epilepsy and mental retardation are other features.

Other manifestations include facial adenoma sebaceum (as in this patient), cutaneous cafe-au-lait spots, shagreen and ash leaf patches, subungal fibromas, ocular phakomas, renal angiomyolipomas, lung fibrosis, and cardiac rhabdomyomas.

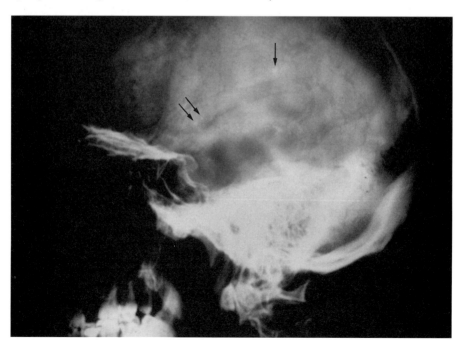

Fig. 1a   Lateral skull radiograph in tuberous sclerosis.

Question 2

A 37-year-old chronic alcoholic was admitted with a history of intermittent episodes of loss of consciousness. These were ascribed to alcoholic binges. However, an unenhanced computed tomography (CT) brain scan was performed on this admission. What is the diagnosis?

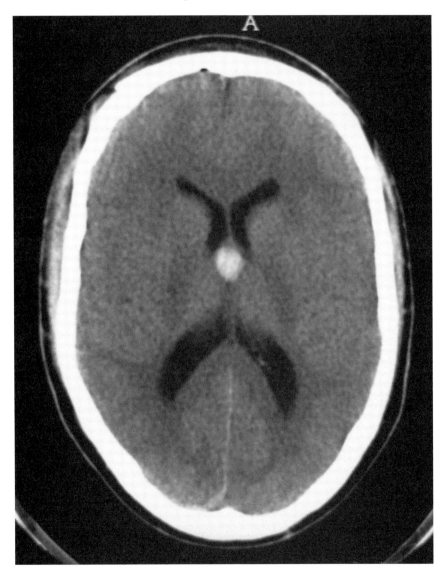

Fig. 2

Answer 2: Colloid cyst of the third ventricle

Findings: A dense, rounded mass is seen in the position of the foramen of Monro causing minor hydrocephalus of the lateral ventricles.

Although these cysts may present with progressive mental deterioration secondary to chronic intracranial hypertension they more often present with acute episodes of loss of consciousness. This is due to the cyst acting intermittently as a ball valve with obstruction of the foramen of Monro. The cysts are thought to be of ependymal origin and are almost always located at the anterosuperior portion of the third ventricle. They occur in young adults with a male predominance. The differential is from a meningioma, ependymoma, or an aneurysm, all of which enhance with intravenous contrast unlike a colloid cyst. Management options include treatment of the hydrocephalus itself (via a ventricular shunt), cyst aspiration, or the definitive treatment of surgical excision.

Question 3

This 75-year-old lady, on anticoagulants for a prosthetic mitral valve, presented to her general practitioner with a 3-week history of headaches and blurred vision. The contrast-enhanced CT brain scan is shown. What is the diagnosis?

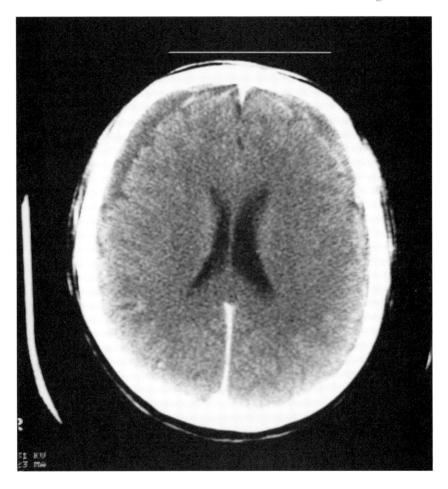

Fig. 3

Answer 3: Chronic bilateral subdural haematomas

Findings: Bilateral low density crescentic shaped haematomas are seen overlying the frontoparietal cortices.

In acute haemorrhage, blood appears white (high density) relative to the normal brain and remains so for 1 week. After approximately 3 weeks it is less dense (as in this case). Therefore there is an interim period of about 2 weeks when the haematoma is isodense with brain and so difficult to diagnose. A contrast enhanced scan may be helpful as cortical vessels in the enveloping membrane are seen to be displaced away from the cranial vault (noted on this scan).

When bilateral subdural haematomas are present, mass effect is evidenced by effacement of the sulci and ventricular compression such that ventricular size is smaller than expected for age. In unilateral subdural haematomas mass effect is indicated by midline shift, ipsilateral ventricular compression, or contralateral ventricular dilatation. Mass effect occurs secondary to the osmotic effect of blood and leads to raised intracranial pressure.

Subdural haematomas result from leakage of blood from torn fragile cortical veins. Predisposing factors are old age, alcoholism, epilepsy, and coagulopathies. Clinical features are altered conscious level, cognitive deficit, and headache which may fluctuate. Neurological signs may be ill defined. A large proportion give no history of trauma.

Question 4

This is the unenhanced CT brain scan of a 34-year-old woman who was found unconscious. What is the diagnosis?

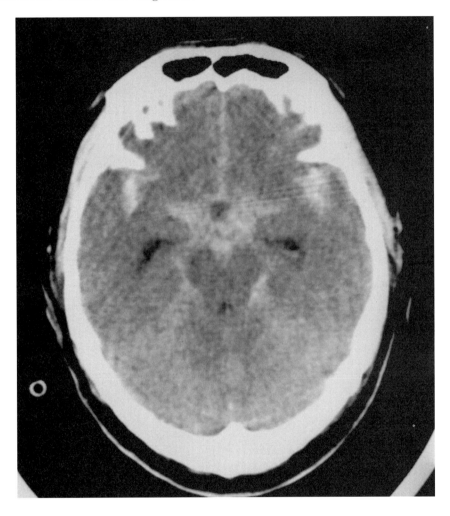

Fig. 4

Answer 4: Subarachnoid haemorrhage

Findings: The CT brain scan shows acute haemorrhage (high attenuation material) in the subarachnoid cisterns around the midbrain and in the sylvian fissures.

Causes of subarachnoid haemorrhage are:

(1) saccular (berry) aneurysm 70%; (2) arteriovenous malformation 10%;
(3) no cause identified 10 to 15%.

Rare causes are: coagulopathies, mycotic aneurysms, bacterial meningitis, trauma, spinal vascular malformation, haemorrhagic tumour, and vasculitides.

Figure 4a shows a carotid angiogram of the patient demonstrating a berry aneurysm of the anterior communicating artery (arrow) the neck of which may be surgically clipped.

The sites of saccular aneurysms are:

(1) anterior communicating artery (junction with anterior cerebral artery) 30%;
(2) posterior communicating artery (junction with internal carotid artery) 25%;
(3) middle cerebral artery (branching point) 21%;
(4) terminal carotid artery 13%;
(5) basilar and posterior inferior cerebellar arteries 3%.

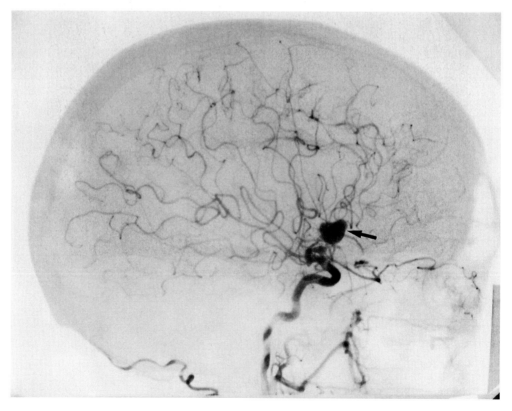

Fig. 4a   Carotid angiogram demonstrating a berry aneurysm of the anterior communicating artery.

Question 5

This is a gadolinium enhanced axial T1 weighted image from an MR study on a 24-year-old woman with hearing loss and tinitus. What is the diagnosis?

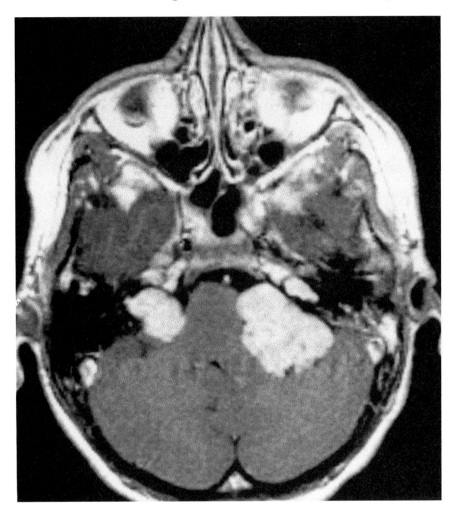

Fig. 5

Answer 5: Bilateral acoustic neuromas

Findings: There are large bilateral cerebello-pontine angle (CPA) masses (high signal) extending out from the internal auditory canals which show intense enhancement. The lesions were moderately hypointense on the precontrast T1 weighted images and hyper-intense on the T2W images (not shown).

Typically, an acoustic neuroma is a solitary lesion in an adult, nearly always taking origin from the vestibular branch of the eighth cranial nerve. It is most common in the fifth and sixth decades. The tumour may occur as part of neurofibromatosis (NF) and bilateral acoustic neuromas are typical of type 2 NF. The tumour typically originates just within the internal auditory canal and grows into the CPA of the posterior fossa. Here it may compress the trigeminal and facial, and less frequently the glossopharyngeal and vagus nerves. As the tumour enlarges, the pons, lateral medulla, and cerebellum are compressed and obstructive hydrocephalus may occur. The most common early symptom is hearing loss with headache; disturbed balance and unsteady gait are less common. Examination shows vestibular and cochlear nerve involvement in >95%.

Imaging is central to the diagnosis of acoustic neuroma. CT may be used, but is not as sensitive as MRI which will identify nearly all tumours. Examinations show a strongly enhancing mass lesion expanding from the internal auditory canal into the CPA.

The differential for CPA masses is acoustic neuroma (75%), meningioma (10%), epidermoid (5%) and vascular lesions, metastases, and other primary intracranial tumours. The treatment of choice of acoustic neuroma is surgical excision. In most cases, the facial nerve can be preserved and in some cases the cochlear nerve.

Question 6

This 26-year-old man's conscious level deteriorated following a head injury at an outdoor music festival. What is the diagnosis?

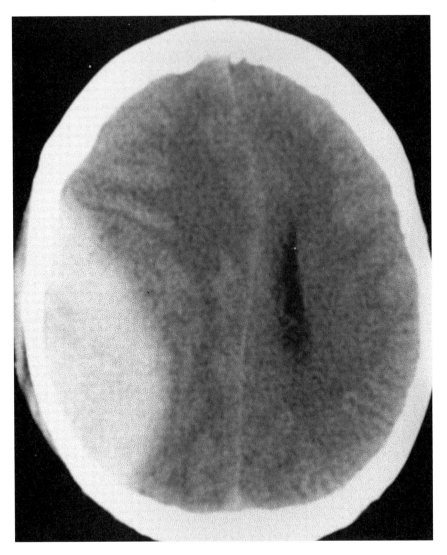

Fig. 6

Answer 6: Acute right extradural haematoma

Findings: There is a biconvex collection of acute haemorrhage in the right parietal region which has associated mass effect as shown by midline shift to the left and compression of the right lateral ventricle.

An extradural haematoma is most commonly associated with a skull fracture (75%) following a head injury. Classically a temporal fracture (which may be identified on CT bony window settings) results in laceration of the middle meningeal artery. Blood strips the dura off the inner table of the skull but as the dura is tightly bound down at the suture margins a rapid rise in intracranial pressure may occur. An extradural haematoma is thus biconvex in shape whereas a subdural haematoma is concavoconvex, as the latter has no anatomical constraints. Typically there is transient loss of consciousness at the time of the head injury followed by a lucid interval and then after a variable time period (which may be a few hours) deterioration in conscious level occurs. This is a neurosurgical emergency requiring urgent drainage.

Question 7

This is a T1 weighted sagittal image from a MR study of the cervical spine performed on a 34-year-old man complaining of upper limb weakness. What is the radiological diagnosis and what findings may be elicited on full neurological examination?

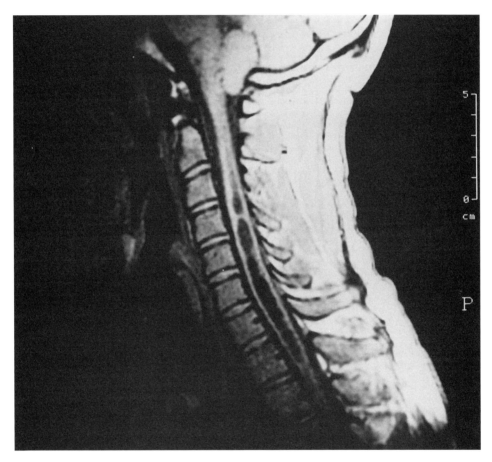

Fig. 7

Answer 7: Syringomyelia

Findings: There is a fusiform region of low signal seen within the cervical portion of the spinal cord in keeping with syringomyelia. Additionally, an Arnold–Chiari type 1 malformation is seen, with herniation of the cerebellar tonsils through the foramen magnum.

Syringomyelia is cavitation of the central canal of the spinal cord, usually located in the cervical region. Commonly there is chronic, progressive degeneration seen clinically as dissociated brachial amyotrophy and sensory loss. Clinical onset is usually insidious. Exacerbations may follow physical strain.

Classical findings on examination are segmental (usually bilateral) wasting and weakness of the hands and arms with diminished reflexes. Dissociated sensory loss is present in the upper limbs with loss of pain and thermal sensation (due to destruction of the decussating spinothalamic nerve axons) and preservation of light touch, vibration, and joint position (carried by the dorsal column fibres). The legs show spastic weakness as a result of corticospinal tract involvement. Other, less common, features are Horner's syndrome and pain.

Diagnosis is often clear from the clinical picture. The investigation of choice for demonstration of the extent of a syrinx, or any related pathology, is MRI. Alternatively, contrast myelography with delayed CT imaging may be used.

Question 8

What is the diagnosis?

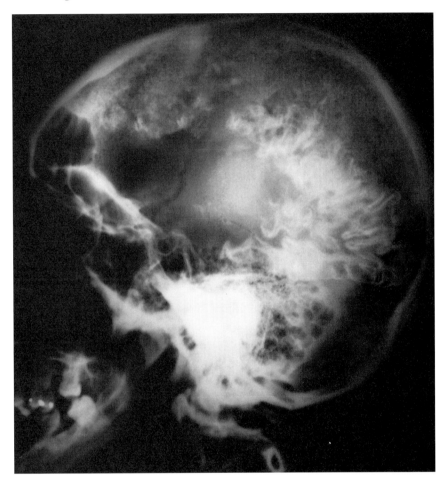

Fig. 8

Answer 8: Sturge–Weber syndrome

Findings: Serpiginous 'tram-track' calcifications are seen over the fronto-parietal-occipital cortex.

The Sturge–Weber syndrome (encephalotrigeminal angiomatosis) is one of the neuroecto-dermal syndromes. There may be a genetic predisposition but familial occurrence is exceptional. The syndrome consists of a congenital facial port-wine naevus (capillary haemangioma) involving the area supplied by the trigeminal nerve (usually first and second divisions). There is an associated ipsilateral venous haemangioma of the pia mater which is most commonly located over the parietal cortex. If the facial naevus is in the area supplied by the first division of the trigeminal nerve, the intracranial lesion is usually over the occipital lobe and a naevus of the second division is most commonly associated with a pial angioma of the parietal region. Cortical hemiatrophy occurs beneath the meningeal angioma due to anoxia (steal) and epilepsy, hemiparesis, and mental retardation are common features. The gyriform pattern seen on the plain skull radiograph corresponds to calcification of the underlying atrophic cerebral cortex and not of the angioma itself. Angiomas may be seen in other organs, including the kidneys, spleen, ovaries, intestines, adrenals, thyroid, pancreas, heart, thymus, and lungs.

Question 9

This 26-year-old man presented with a grand mal fit. What is the diagnosis on the pre- and postcontrast CT brain scans?

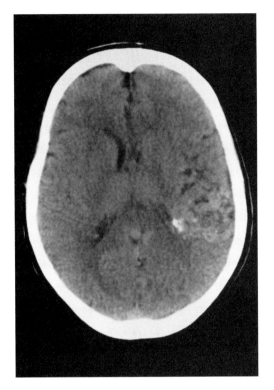

Fig. 9a

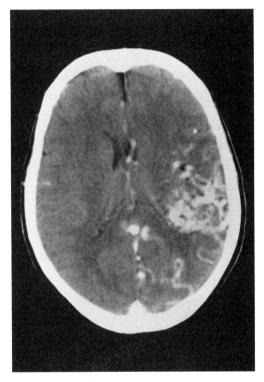

Fig. 9b

Answer 9: *Cerebral arteriovenous malformation (AVM)*

Findings: On the unenhanced image (Fig. 9a) there are scattered calcifications in the left parietal lobe with no associated haemorrhage. Serpiginous black areas are seen which, following intravenous contrast medium (Fig. 9b), enhance and represent an arteriovenous malformation.

Cerebral arteriovenous malformations are congenital and are the commonest vascular anomaly of the central nervous system. Twenty per cent present by 20 years of age and 80% by the end of the fourth decade. Presentation is with headaches, fits, progressive neurological deficit (50%), or acute cerebral haemorrhage (50%). They are mainly supratentorial (80 to 90%) with the parietal lobe being the commonest site. The vascular supply is via pial branches of the internal carotid artery in 80% of supratentorial AVMs and 50% of posterior fossa AVMs. The skull radiograph may show ring-like calcifications with thinning of the skull at contact points with the AVM and prominent vascular grooves on the inner table of the skull. Angiography is necessary to identify feeding vessels that may be amenable to embolization. Other forms of treatment are surgery or radiotherapy. Complications include haemorrhage, especially on the venous side, and infarction. Subarachnoid haemorrhage is due to AVMs in approximately 10% of cases. Haemorrhage from an AVM is associated with a 10% mortality and a 30% morbidity. There is a 2 to 3% yearly chance of haemorrhage which increases to 6% in the year following a first bleed and 25% in the year after a second bleed.

Question 10

This is a gadolinium enhanced T1 weighted sagittal MR image in the region of the brainstem (B), third ventricle, corpus callosum (C), and sphenoid sinus (S). This 19-year-old girl complained of secondary amenorrhoea. Describe the lesion seen and what is the most likely diagnosis?

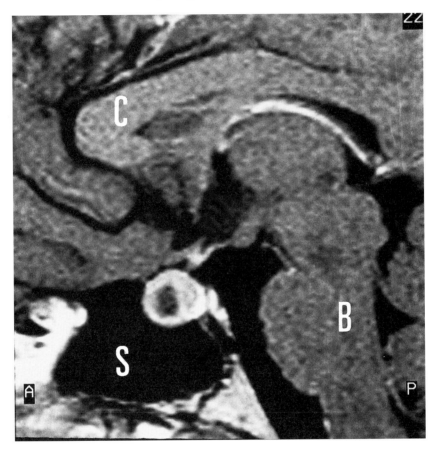

Fig. 10

Answer 10: Prolactin secreting pituitary adenoma

Findings: There is a 1 cm unenhancing, partly cystic mass in the pituitary fossa (Fig. 10a, paired arrows). The normal pituitary tissue is seen to enhance around the adenoma. The optic chiasma is not compressed (curved arrow).

Tumours of the anterior pituitary (adenohypophysis) may be chromophobe, acidophil, or basophil. Chromophobe and acidophil tumours may secrete prolactin, GH, or TSH. Basophil tumours produce ACTH, LH, and FSH. Prolactinomas account for 30% of all pituitary tumours. Tumours less than 10 mm are microadenomata. As a tumour grows, it compresses the normal pituitary and extends out of the sella superiorly to involve the optic pathway. The clinical presentation is variable. Visual and endocrine features are the most common causes of presentation. Headache is found in 50% patients with a macroadenoma. The visual defect is usually a degree of bitemporal hemianopia, but early presentation may be with bitemporal upper field quadrantanopia. Less common clinical features include: ocular palsies (5 to 10%, from cavernous sinus invasion), seizures, diabetes insipidus, and cerebrospinal fluid rhinorrhoea.

MRI is the most sensitive method of demonstrating a pituitary tumour. Tumour extent is of practical importance because surgery is easier and more successful if there is no extension beyond the sella. Trans-sphenoidal surgical excision of the tumour is usually curative. Bromocriptine (a dopamine agonist) may be used to control prolactin and GH-secreting tumours. In GH-secreting tumours octreotide (a somatostatin analogue) can also be used. Radiotherapy is used when medical and surgical management fails.

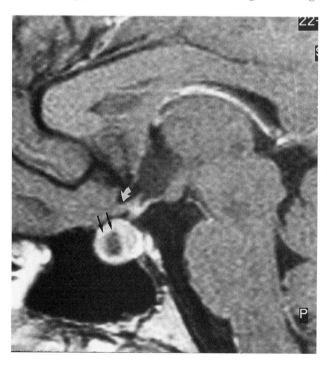

Fig. 10a Sagittal MRI showing a prolactin secreting pituitary adenoma.

Question 11

This contrast enhanced T1 weighted sagittal MR image is from a study performed on a 28-year-old woman who developed headaches 2 days postpartum and was found to have bilateral papilloedema. Describe the radiological findings and what is the diagnosis?

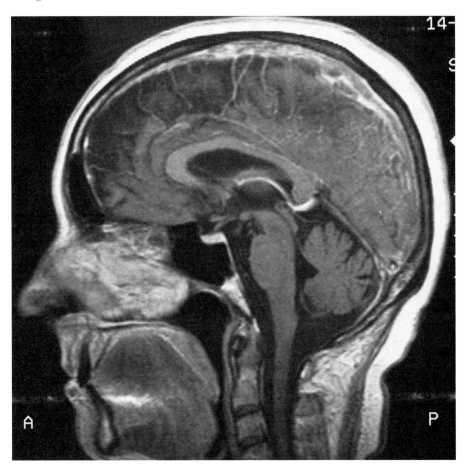

Fig. 11

Answer 11: Superior sagittal sinus thrombosis (SST)

Findings: The superior sagittal sinus contains irregular intermediate signal material (thrombus, arrows on Fig. 11a) surrounded by high signal from gadolinium enhancement. Normally the superior sagittal sinus appears as a flow void (black) as no magnetic signal is obtained from flowing blood.

The process of SST usually starts as non-occlusive thrombus formation in the superior sagittal sinus, which progresses to occlusion and extension into the cerebral veins. Involvement of the cerebral veins results in the formation of petechial haemorrhages and venous infarction. Conditions predisposing to SST include:

- pregnancy, puerperium, and oral contraceptive pill
- dehydration
- local tumour
- drugs.
- infection
- hypercoagulable states
- trauma

The presenting features are variable and a high degree of clinical suspicion is required if under-diagnosis is to be avoided. Imaging is central to the confirmation of the diagnosis. Patients may have headache and vomiting; neurological symptoms are variable. On examination, bilateral sixth nerve palsy and papilloedema may be found. Fever is absent unless there is underlying infection. Lumbar puncture is normal apart from elevation of the cerebrospinal fluid pressure.

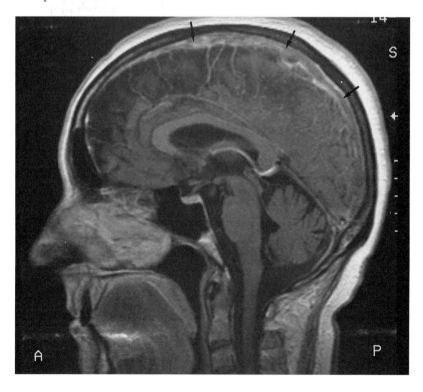

Fig. 11a Sagittal MRI showing superior sagittal sinus thrombosis.

Question 12

This is an axial image from a T2 weighted MR study of a 42-year-old woman who presented with a 12-year history of variable sensory deficit. What is the diagnosis?

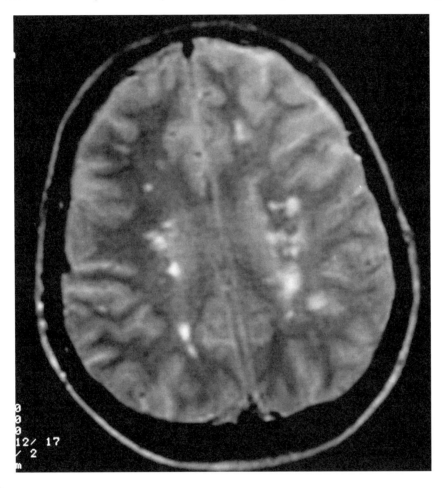

Fig. 12

Answer 12: Multiple sclerosis (MS)

Findings: Multiple areas of high signal are seen in both corona radiata.

MS is the most frequently found chronic inflammatory demyelinating disease. MS has to be differentiated from acute disseminated encephalomyelitis which does not have the remitting and relapsing features of MS. Pathologically, myelin degeneration leads to scar (plaque) formation. The aetiology is uncertain. Incidence varies with location, from 1 in 100 000 in equatorial areas to up to 1 in 1000 in northern Europe and North America. People migrating from a high incidence to a low incidence region take with them some of the risk of their birth place. There is a familial tendency to MS, with 15% of affected individuals having an affected relative. The male:female incidence is 1:2 and age of onset is between 20 and 40 years in 66%.

Characteristically, the clinical features are of focal neurological deficits which remit to a variable degree and recur over a period of many years. The specific neurological features vary, but reflect lesions which affect the optic nerves, spinal cord, and brain. In the acute phase, 50% show an increase in monocytes in the cerebrospinal fluid. Electrophoresis of cerebrospinal fluid will demonstrate abnormally increased gamma globulin (oligoclonal bands) in 90% of all cases of MS.

Imaging to confirm the diagnosis of MS is best performed with MR. Ovoid periventricular plaques, orientated perpendicular to the long axis of the brain and ventricles, are seen in 85% (Dawson's fingers). Greater than 50% of patients show involvement of the corpus callosum. The posterior fossa is a less frequent site of involvement, with lesions seen in 10% (more common in adolescents).

Question 13

This 67-year-old woman underwent a CT brain scan having been found at home unrousable. What are the CT findings? What causes are there for this pathology?

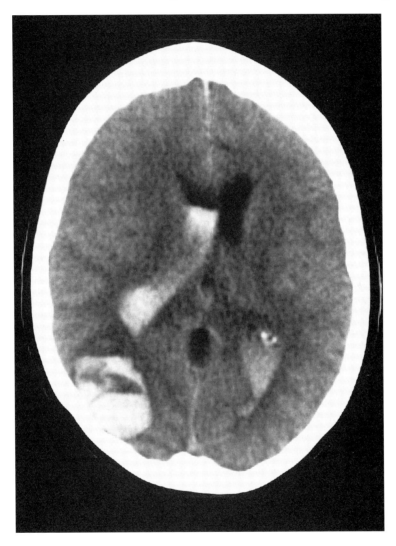

Fig. 13

Answer 13: Cerebral haematoma with intraventricular extension

Findings: There is a 4 cm, mixed attenuation lesion in the right occipital region. Two fluid levels are seen due to settling of the blood products within the haematoma, the higher attenuation portion is dependent. There is associated midline shift, indicating mass effect from the haematoma. There is also blood in the ventricular system and there is effacement of the sulci and early enlargement of the ventricular system, in keeping with evolving hydrocephalus.

Aetiology of cerebral haematoma:

(1)   aneurysm (33%);
(2)   hypertension (33%)—most often located in the basal ganglia or thalamus (75%);
(3)   arteriovenous malformation (10%);
(4)   trauma;
(5)   haemorrhagic infarction;
(6)   bleeding into tumour;
(7)   hypocoagulable state.

The features of a cerebral haematoma on non-enhanced CT vary with its age. In the first 24 hours an homogeneous high attenuation lesion with an irregular but well defined periphery is seen. As the haematoma consolidates, layering is often seen and its attenuation decreases so that there is a stage between 3 and 10 weeks when it is isointense with surrounding brain and has an associated hypointense rim. During resolution, osmotic fluid uptake may cause the cerebral haematoma to appear hypointense compared with surrounding brain.

CT is superior to MRI in the identification of acute haemorrhage as acute blood may be isointense to brain on MRI.

Question 14

This 48-year-old man presented with fits that were unresponsive to medical therapy. What is the most likely diagnosis on this unenhanced CT brain?

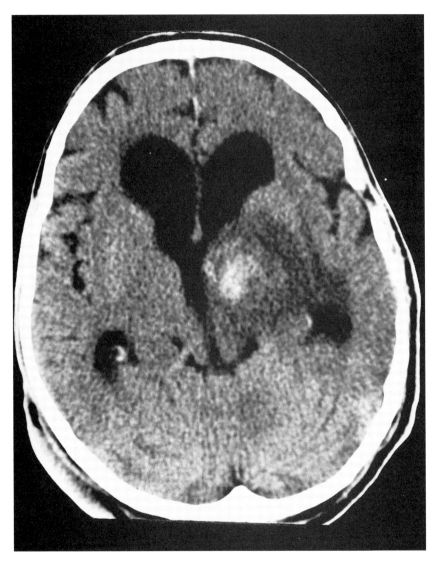

Fig. 14

Answer 14: *Primary cerebral malignant tumour (oligodendroglioma)*

Findings: A 4-cm mass is seen in the left basal ganglia which is predominantly low attenuation, but has a high attenuation central region. The high attenuation is due to calcification on this unenhanced scan (haemorrhage would appear similar). There is mass effect with midline shift to the right. Hydrocephalus is indicated by dilated frontal horns.

In patients with oligodendroglioma, the first symptom in over 50% is focal or generalized seizures. There is often a gap of many years before additional symptoms develop. Raised intracranial pressure is present in 15% at presentation. Findings on examination vary with the site of the tumour. Oligodendrogliomas are uncommon intracranial tumours (5% of primary intracranial neoplasms). They most commonly occur in the cerebral hemispheres, with a predilection for the frontal lobes.

CT shows a rounded, hypodense lesion with mass effect in 75% of cases, oedema in only 50% of low grade lesions, and more than minimal enhancement in only 25% of cases. Calcification is seen in 70 to 90%. Other calcified intracranial masses include:

- craniopharyngioma
- astrocytoma
- choroid plexus papilloma
- meningioma
- ependymoma
- aneurysm.

Question 15

This 78-year-old lady was brought to hospital with an acute hemiparesis. What is the diagnosis?

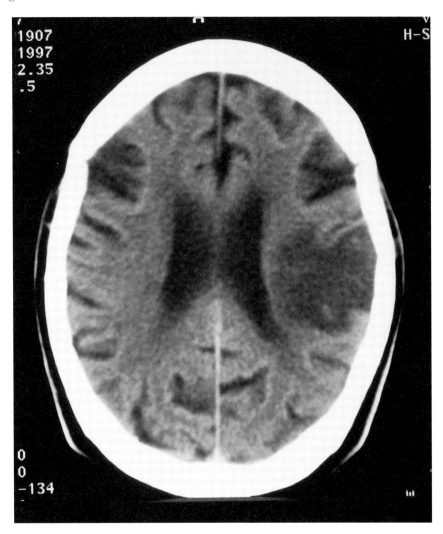

Fig. 15

Answer 15: Cerebral infarct

Findings: There is a hypodense, wedge-shaped lesion in the territory of the left middle cerebral artery. The base of the wedge is at the cortical surface and there is effacement of sulci.

Ischaemic cerebral infarction may be broadly divided into thrombotic and embolic. Most cerebrovascular accidents can be ascribed to atherothrombosis. The atheromatous plaques formed have a predilection for branch points and are most common at the carotid bifurcation, junction of the vertebral arteries, and middle cerebral artery bifurcation. In 75%, a major thrombotic event is preceded by transient ischaemic episodes or minor symptoms. Rarely are embolic and haemorrhagic cerebral events heralded by a prodromal episode.

Embolic cerebral infarction most often has a cardiac basis (e.g. atrial fibrillation, mural thrombus following myocardial infarction, bacterial endocarditis, and prosthetic valves).

In patients at risk of cerebral infarction, echocardiography and carotid Doppler ultrasound may be used to identify treatable lesions. MRI is more sensitive than CT in the detection of cerebral infarction. Depending on the sequences used, MRI is positive as early as 1 to 6 hours. With CT, detection varies with lesion type; 80% of infarcts involving the cortex will be identified, while only 50% of those affecting the basal ganglia or posterior fossa will be demonstrated. CT sensitivity also varies with the time from onset of clinical symptoms. On the day of the event, 50% of infarcts will be identified, while 75% will be seen at day 10. CT performed early is useful in excluding a haemorrhagic component so that aspirin may be commenced.

Question 16

What lesion is present on the unenhanced CT scan of this 70-year-old lady who presented with headaches?

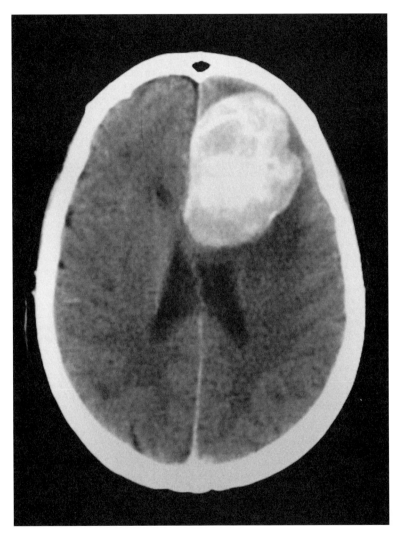

Fig. 16

Answer 16: Meningioma with heavy calcification

Findings: Arising from the falx cerebri there is a well defined, densely calcified mass. There is mass effect with midline shift to the right, effacement of sulci, and associated oedema. Compression of the left frontal horn is also seen.

Meningiomas comprise 15% of primary intracranial tumours and have a F:M ratio of 2:1. The peak age of presentation is 45 years (range 30 to 75).

Meningiomas are the commonest radiation-induced tumours of the central nervous system. Lesions are most commonly located at the convexity of the lateral aspect of the cerebral hemisphere (30%), parasagittal (25%), sphenoid wing/ middle cranial fossa (20%), and spinal canal (10%).

Presenting features vary. Many meningiomas are found incidentally. Small lesions lying around the floor of the third ventricle may present early; while frontoparietal lesions may be large by the time of diagnosis. Focal seizures are often an early sign.

CT, MRI, or angiography may all be used to establish the diagnosis. The non-invasive nature of CT and MRI makes them favourable. CT shows a smooth-edged, iso/hyperdense mass which abuts a meningeal surface and most enhance strongly with intravenous contrast. The amount of associated oedema is usually less than that seen with primary and secondary malignant cerebral tumours. Calcification is seen in 20% and hyperostosis of the adjacent bone in 20% of cases.

Surgical excision results in a permanent cure in the majority of patients with a readily accessible tumour. The en plaque type of tumour, particularly in the parasellar region or on the lesser wing of the sphenoid, may invade bone and is technically more difficult to excise. This type of tumour may be treated with radiotherapy.

Question 17

A 53-year-old man presented with a rapid deterioration in neurological function. The MR scan shows a gadolinium enhanced T1 weighted axial section through the posterior fossa, temporal lobes, and orbits. What is the most likely diagnosis?

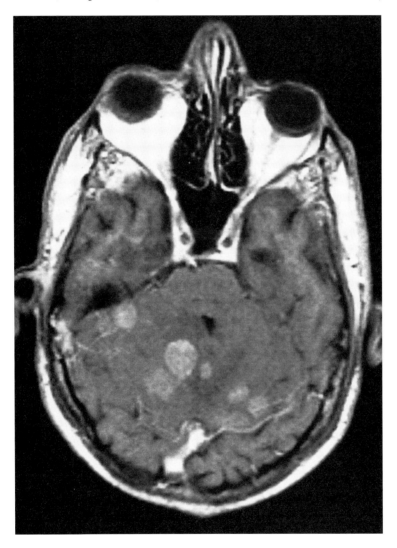

Fig. 17

Answer 17: Cerebellar metastases

Findings: Multiple rounded lesions of higher signal intensity than surrounding neural tissue are seen in the cerebellum. The lesions were isointense with brain on T2 and precontrast T1 weighted images, but were identified by virtue of their mass effect and surrounding oedema. Additional lesions were found in the cerebral hemispheres.

The clinical presentation of cerebral metastases is similar to that of a cerebral primary tumour and is variable. Symptoms are progressive and may include: headache, seizures, motor/ sensory or cerebellar dysfunction, and mental or behavioural abnormalities. On examination there may be raised intracranial pressure or focal neurological deficit. Metastases account for nearly 25% of intracranial tumours. Multiple deposits at first presentation are seen in 66% of cases. The majority of lesions are found in the supratentorial space and when they are multiple, they are usually of varied size. Five primary tumours account for 95% of metastases:

(1)   bronchial (50%, rarely squamous);
(2)   breast (15%);
(3)   gastrointestinal (15%);
(4)   hypernephroma (10%);
(5)   melanoma (10%).

Haemorrhagic metastases account for less than 5% of deposits and are most commonly from melanoma, oat cell lung carcinoma, renal cell carcinoma, choriocarcinoma, or thyroid carcinoma. MRI is more sensitive than CT, but the lesion characteristics are similar on the two modalities. The deposits are usually solid, with surrounding (vasogenic) oedema exceeding tumour volume, and enhance strongly. With larger tumours, the enhancement may be ring-like.

Question 18

These sagittal T2 weighted sections are from a MR study performed on a 63-year-old man with a 3-month history of back pain and 2 weeks of worsening numbness and weakness of both legs. What abnormalities are shown? What is the diagnosis?

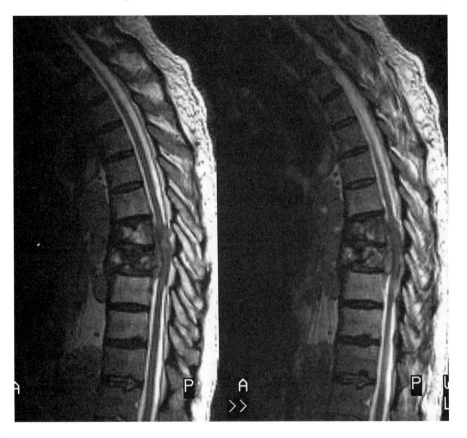

Fig. 18

Answer 18: Malignant spinal cord compression

Findings: The T8 and T9 vertebral bodies are destroyed, with heterogeneous signal and loss of height. The intervertebral discs are spared. There is a large associated soft tissue mass which extends from T6 to 10 anteriorly and into the spinal canal posteriorly, where there is compression of the spinal cord. Signal abnormality is seen in several other vertebral bodies, and there is a further large soft tissue mass lying anterior to T12 to L2, in keeping with widespread malignant disease. The large soft tissue masses lying anterior to the vertebral column, and the sparing of the intervertebral discs, make a malignant cause much more likely than an infective one.

Metastases to the spine are most commonly from; breast, prostate, lung, kidney, and melanoma.

The clinical features of malignant cord compression vary. There may be symptoms and signs related to the primary lesion. The secondary deposit usually causes pain. The neurological features depend on the level of the lesion and the degree of cord compression.

Question 19

This is a T2 weighted sagittal image of a 37-year-old woman who presented with pain over the right scapular region, radiating down the arm to the index finger. What is the cause of the pain and what findings may be elicited on neurological examination?

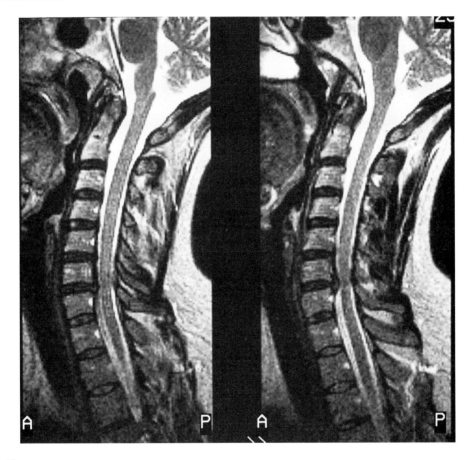

Fig. 19

Answer 19: *Prolapse of cervical intervertebral disc*

Findings: There is disc space narrowing at the C6/7 level with disc protrusion into the spinal canal. Comparison with simultaneous T1 weighted sagittal and T2 weighted axial images showed the disc prolapse to be right paracentral (not shown).

Protrusion of the intervertebral disc centrally compromises the spinal cord. Protrusion posterolaterally causes root compression. The cervical roots most commonly affected by a disc protrusion are C7 (70%), C6 (20%), and C5 and C8 (10%).

C6 root compression (by a C5 to 6 lateral protrusion) results in pain along the trapezius ridge to the shoulder tip with radiation to the anterior part of the arm, the lateral aspect of the forearm, and the thumb. Paraesthesia and tenderness are found in the same distribution. Weakness of elbow flexion is found, with diminished biceps and supinator reflexes.

C7 compression causes pain (with paraesthesias and tenderness) over the scapula, medial axilla, and pectoral region with radiation to the posterolateral part of the arm, the posterior part of the forearm, and the index/ middle fingers. Weakness is mainly of elbow extension, with the triceps tendon jerk diminished.

C8 compression gives pain, paraesthesias, and tenderness along the medial forearm and ring and little fingers. Weakness is of the muscles supplied by the ulnar nerve.

There is poor correlation between the plain radiograph findings of long-standing disc-space narrowing with bony changes and the severity of the clinical picture. The diagnosis is best confirmed by MRI.

Conservative treatment of a root compression syndrome, with traction or a collar, is often successful.

RESPIRATORY DISEASE

Question 20

This is a chest radiograph of a 25-year-old female with chronic sputum production. What is the diagnosis?

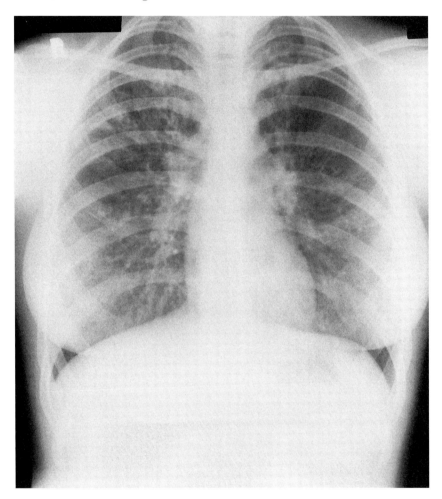

Fig. 20

Answer 20: Bronchiectasis

Findings: The chest radiograph demonstrates cystic bronchiectasis (ring shadows are seen, particularly in the right upper lobe) with lung hyperinflation in a patient with cystic fibrosis. Bilateral hilar lymphadenopathy is also present. Bronchial wall thickening, appearing like tramlines, is seen in the right perihilar region.

Bronchography was used for the diagnosis but because of the high incidence of adverse effects it is no longer used. High resolution CT (HRCT) is now performed with 1 to 2 mm slices every 10 mm through the lungs. The features of bronchiectasis on HRCT are:

(1) dilated bronchi with thickened walls such that they are bigger than their accompanying pulmonary artery, known as the signet ring sign (Fig. 20a, straight arrow);
(2) crowding of the dilated bronchi (Fig. 20a, open arrow head);
(3) mucus plugging (Fig. 20a, curved arrows) and fluid levels within the bronchi;
(4) bronchi seen in the peripheral one-third of the lung, where they are not normally seen, reflecting bronchial wall thickening and dilatation.

Causes of bronchiectasis are:

(1) local—lobar collapse resulting from inhaled foreign body, inhalational pneumonia, tuberculosis, or bronchial carcinoma;
(2) generalized:
    (a) childhood infections—whooping cough, measles, or bronchiolitis;
    (b) cystic fibrosis;
    (c) congenital structural defects—Kartagener's syndrome (bronchiectasis with immotile cilia, dextrocardia, or situs inversus and sinusitis) or Williams–Campbell syndrome (bronchial cartilage deficiency);
    (d) allergic bronchopulmonary aspergillosis (proximal bronchiectasis);
    (e) immune deficiency states, e.g. hypogammaglobulinaemia.

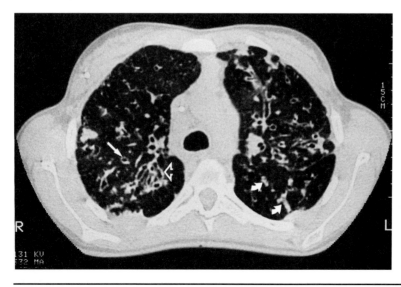

Fig. 20a High resolution CT (HRCT) demonstrating bronchiectasis.

Question 21

This 32-year-old man presented with a 6-month history of exertional dyspnoea and intermittent haemoptysis. Investigations revealed an iron deficiency anaemia. His father had died of a cerebrovascular accident at the age of 40. What is the diagnosis and how would you confirm it?

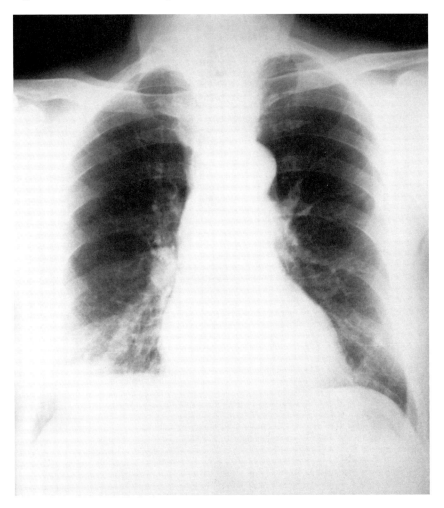

Fig. 21

Answer 21: Pulmonary arteriovenous malformation (AVM) associated with Osler–Weber–Rendu syndrome

Findings: A well-defined, lobulated mass is seen in the right lower zone with prominent associated hilar vessels and cord-like bands between them (feeding and draining vessels).

The diagnosis is confirmed by contrast enhanced CT (Fig. 21a, arrow) which also identifies the feeding vessels. Pulmonary angiography may be required prior to therapy.

Pulmonary AVMs may be congenital or acquired. The congenital variant is commoner and may be an isolated finding in 40% and multiple in 33% of cases. Approximately 50% of patients with an AVM have hereditary haemorrhagic telangiectasia (Osler–Weber–Rendu syndrome) but only 15% of patients with this disease have AVMs. Other features of hereditary haemorrhagic telangiectasia are family history, gastrointestinal bleeds, epistaxis, and telangectasia of the skin/ mucosal membranes.

Clinical features include presentation in the 30 to 40 age group, exertional dyspnoea, cyanosis, clubbing, and a bruit heard over the lesion. Patients may be asymptomatic and the chest radiograph normal. Complications include cerebrovascular accident and cerebral abscess secondary to paradoxical embolism, haemoptysis, haemothorax, and polycythaemia.

Management may be surgical or embolization with coils.

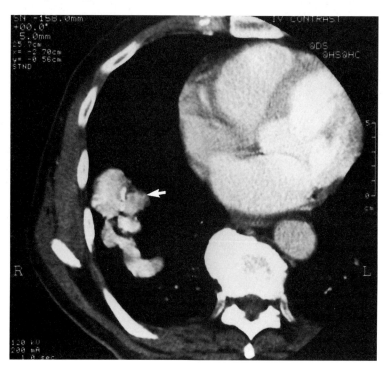

Fig. 21a   Axial enhanced CT chest showing a right pulmonary arteriovenous malformation (arrow).

Question 22

This 65-year-old man presented with a 6-month history of a pain in the left shoulder, which radiated into the arm. What is the diagnosis?

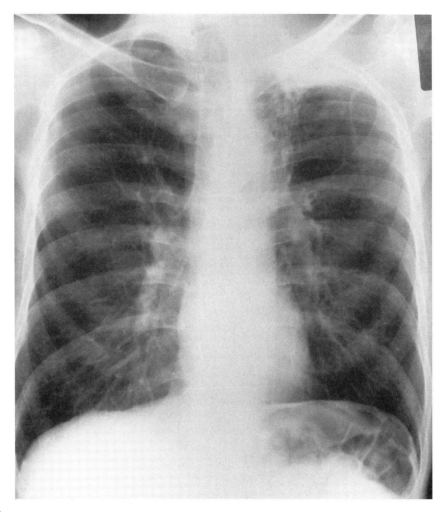

Fig. 22

Answer 22: Pancoast tumour (apical or superior sulcus pulmonary neoplasm)

Findings: There is an opacity in the left apex of the lung associated with destruction of the first, second, and third ribs posteriorly. There is also loss of volume in the left upper lobe with crowding of vessels and bronchi medially and elevation of the left hilum.

The specificity of the Pancoast tumour relates to the clinical presentation; any cell type may be present. The histology is usually squamous cell.

Clinically, pain in the shoulder and arm is due to invasion of the brachial plexus, or the ribs/ vertebral column. If there is invasion of the sympathetic chain, an ipsilateral Horner's syndrome results. Findings on examination vary with the pattern of invasion.

As a result of its position, the lesion may be hard to identify on a CXR. An apical mass is seen in 66% of cases, rib or vertebral destruction being seen in 33%. A high degree of clinical suspicion must be maintained and CT/MRI and biopsy arranged where necessary. MRI has the advantage of superior demonstration of the soft tissue invasion around the brachial plexus and subclavian vessels. Histology is essential.

Question 23

This is a perfusion/ ventilation (V/Q) scan of a 32-year-old lady with acute dyspnoea. The top row shows the perfusion images and the lower row the ventilation images. What is the diagnosis?

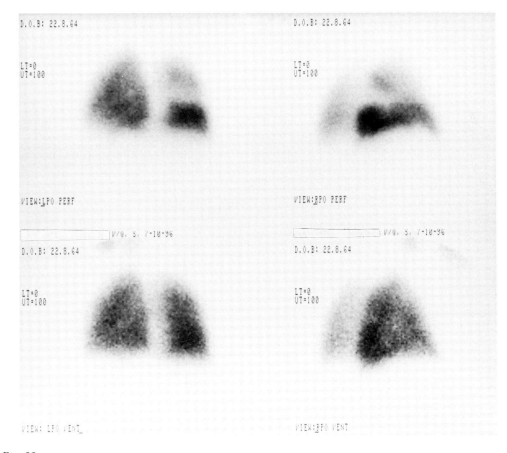

Fig. 23

Answer 23: Pulmonary embolus (PE)

Findings: The V/Q scan shows a large perfusion defect in the right mid and upper zones without a matched ventilatory defect. This represents a major PE affecting the right upper lobe.

Figure 23a shows a CT pulmonary angiogram, at the level of the pulmonary trunk, of another patient. There are filling defects in both basal pulmonary arteries (curved arrows).

The diagnosis is important as the mortality in untreated patients with PE approaches 30% which can be reduced to 8% with treatment. In PE without infarction the CXR is normal in more than a third. Abnormalities may include: atelectasis, a plump or amputated proximal pulmonary artery containing the thrombus within, pulmonary oligaemia distal to the embolus, and 'consolidation' due to the infarct which is pleurally based or pleural effusion. The V/Q scan gives the probability of PE as high, intermediate, or low, and it must therefore be interpreted carefully. It has an inherent weakness in that it does not directly visualize the thrombus. The most sensitive and specific investigation is pulmonary angiography. This should be performed soon after the suspected diagnosis of PE because of the rapid spontaneous resolution that can occur: 10% by 1 day and 50% by 2 weeks. Spiral CT pulmonary angiogram is more sensitive and specific than ventilation/ perfusion (V/Q) scanning and a CXR in diagnosing PE. CT shows the embolus as a filling defect within the contrast enhanced pulmonary artery and is providing a useful alternative to conventional pulmonary angiography. Treatment may be with heparin followed by warfarin. In major PE, a thrombolytic agent may be used. If there is recurrent PE despite adequate anticoagulation or a contraindication to anticoagulation, a vena caval filter can be inserted to prevent further PEs.

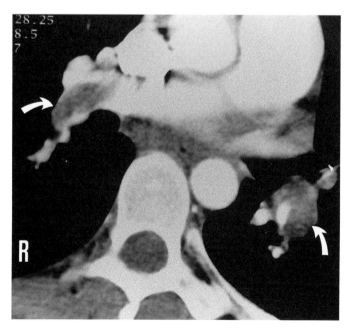

Fig. 23a Spiral CT pulmonary angiogram showing bilateral basal pulmonary arterial emboli (arrows).

Question 24

This 24-year-old man presented with night sweats and weight loss. What is the likely diagnosis?

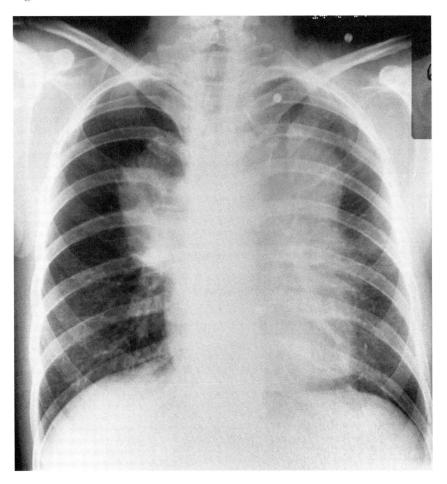

Fig. 24

Answer 24: Hodgkin's disease

Findings: There is a large soft tissue mass which extends bilaterally to obscure the left heart border and the ascending aorta. It must therefore lie in the anterior mediastinum. The hila vessels are clearly seen as is the descending aorta confirming that the mass does not extend posteriorly or into the perihilar regions (they are clearly seen due to the adjacent air/ normal soft tissue interface, i.e. the silhouette sign). Fig. 24a shows an enhanced CT demonstrating the anterior mediastinal lymphadenopathy (curved arrows).

The differential diagnosis of an anterior mediastinal mass includes:

(1) lymphadenopathy—lymphoma, TB;
(2) thymoma—occurs in 15% of patients with myasthenis gravis and 40% of these are malignant and 60% show thymic hyperplasia;
(3) aneurysm of the ascending aorta;
(4) germ cell tumours—for example teratomas and dermoids;
(5) retrosternal goitre (extends into the mediastinum in 1 to 3% of cases) and is associated with tracheal deviation;
(6) pericardial fat pads or cysts;
(7) diaphragmatic humps and hernias;
(8) tortuous inominate artery.

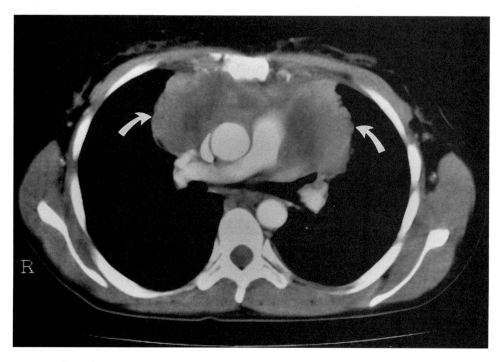

Fig. 24a   Enhanced CT at the level of the pulmonary trunk showing anterior mediastinal lymphadenopathy.

Question 25

This 24-year-old presented with uncontrollable coughing after a fall. What is the diagnosis? What is the cause? What treatment is necessary?

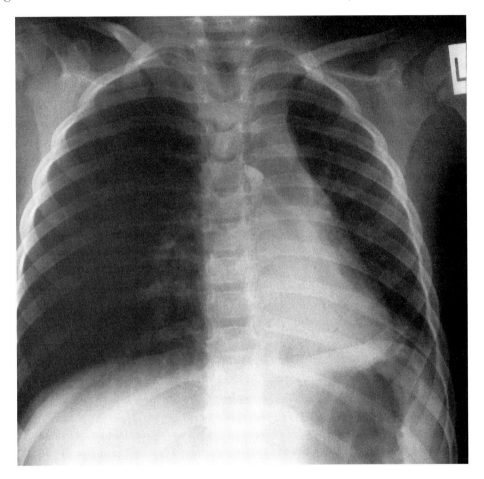

Fig. 25

Answer 25: Left lower lobe collapse (atelectasis)

This is secondary to inhalation of a tooth and bronchoscopy should be undertaken to remove the foreign body.

Findings:

1. Small left hemithorax with a tooth in the left main bronchus.
2. Collapse of the left lower lobe with increased density behind the heart. This has a straight lateral margin due to a depressed oblique fissure. Note the depressed left hilum with vessels converging medially at a point lower than the right hilum.
3. There is an air bronchogram in the left lower lobe implying incomplete proximal obstruction by the tooth.
4. The right lung herniates anteriorly implying loss of volume on the left side.

On a chest radiograph the basic features of collapse are opacity and loss of volume. If there is complete collapse of the left lower lobe against the descending aorta and left hemidiaphragm then these latter structures may not be clearly seen due to loss of the silhouette sign (the silhouette sign is due to the interface between air and a soft tissue structure). Note that complete collapse of the left lower lobe may only be detected by depression of the left hilum.

CT can demonstrate the cause of pulmonary collapse. Fig. 25a shows an axial section from another patient, which shows left lower lobe collapse (straight arrow) secondary to an obstructing tumour (curved arrows) with left atrial invasion (arrowheads).

The most common causes of collapse are pneumonia, mucous plugging (asthma and cystic fibrosis), inhaled foreign body, and bronchial neoplasm.

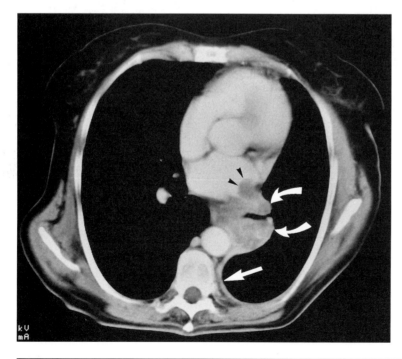

Fig. 25a Axial enhanced CT showing left lower lobe collapse and left atrial invasion due to a bronchial carcinoma.

Question 26

This 68-year-old man presented with haemoptysis and dyspnoea. What is the diagnosis?

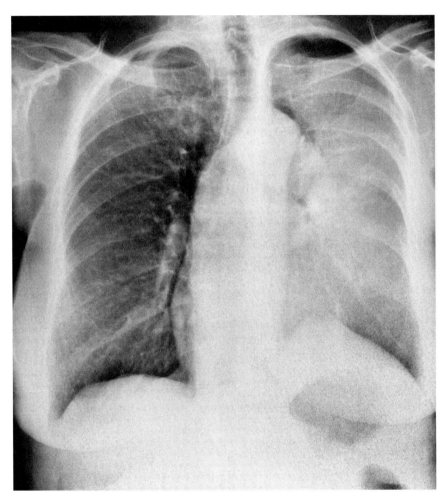

Fig. 26

Answer 26: Left upper lobe collapse secondary to a bronchogenic carcinoma

Findings: There is loss of volume of the left hemithorax, with rib crowding and an elevated left hemidiaphragm. Increased density associated with loss of the left heart border confirms left upper lobe collapse. A left hilar bronchial carcinoma is seen and is responsible for obstruction of the upper lobe bronchus. Air in the left apex is due to the over inflated left lower lobe and there is also herniation of the right upper lobe across the midline.

Figure 26a shows a CT scan at the level of the main pulmonary artery. The central mass surrounding and narrowing the upper lobe bronchus (curved white arrows) can be separated from the distal collapse (straight white arrows). This gives the characteristic sigma shape with a central tumour. Pathological lymphadenopathy (black arrowhead) can be seen. CT is useful in staging bronchial carcinomas and in helping to assess operability.

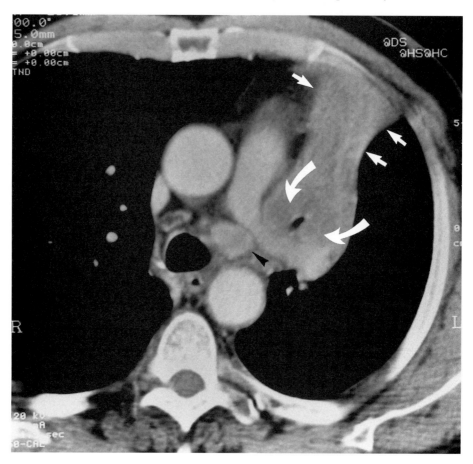

Fig. 26a   CT shows a bronchial carcinoma of the left upper lobe causing distal collapse.

Question 27

This 45-year-old asthmatic presented with cough and pyrexia. What is the diagnosis?

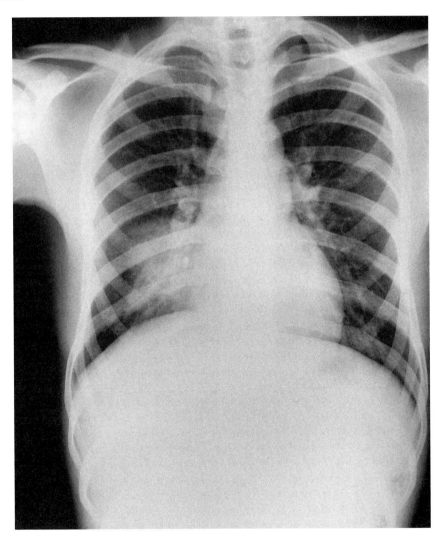

Fig. 27

Answer 27: Right middle lobe collapse—in this patient it was due to mucous plugging

Findings: There is loss of the right heart border with adjacent parenchymal shadowing indicating middle lobe pathology. Collapse is indicated by loss of volume (elevation of the right hemidiaphragm).

A lateral chest radiograph is useful in confirming right middle lobe collapse. There is a wedge-shaped opacity (Fig. 27a) extending anteriorly from the hilum. The lower limit of the collapsed lobe is defined by the oblique fissue (arrows) and its upper extent demarcated by a depressed horizontal fissure (arrowheads).

Physiotherapy or bronchoscopy helps expulsion of the causative mucous plug.

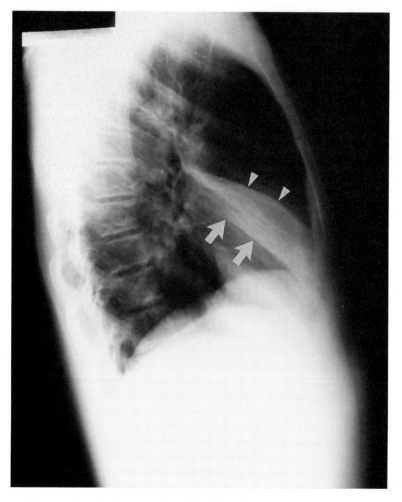

Fig. 27a   Lateral chest radiograph showing right middle lobe collapse.

Question 28

This 24-year-old HIV-positive patient presented with haemoptysis and dyspnoea. What is the most likely diagnosis?

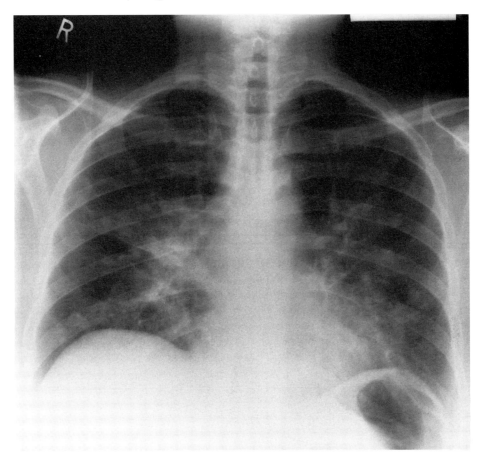

Fig. 28

Answer 28: *Kaposi's sarcoma (KS)*

Findings: There is bilateral nodular shadowing, predominantly in a perihilar distribution, reflecting a bronchocentric distribution of the lesions. There is also diffuse linear interstitial shadowing which reflects the angiomatous type of infiltration of the pulmonary parenchyma.

KS was rare prior to the AIDS epidemic, classically affecting the skin of the lower limbs of elderly men of Jewish and Mediterranean origin. KS is one of the most common malignancies in HIV disease and the cutaneous form is the usual, initial presentation. The lungs are involved in 20% of cases and nodules are common. In the pulmonary form, pleural effusion (30%) and hilar lymphadenopathy (25 to 60%) occur late in the disease.

KS is seen in other forms of immunosuppression apart from HIV and regression is seen with improved immune status. KS has been noted to be commoner in homosexuals than in intravenous drug abusers, suggesting the role of another factor (possibly cytomegalovirus). Therapeutic options include chemotherapy or local radiotherapy but the prognosis is poor.

Question 29

This is the chest radiograph of a 34-year-old man with a 6-month history of increasing breathlessness and intermittent haematemesis. What abnormalities are present and what is the diagnosis?

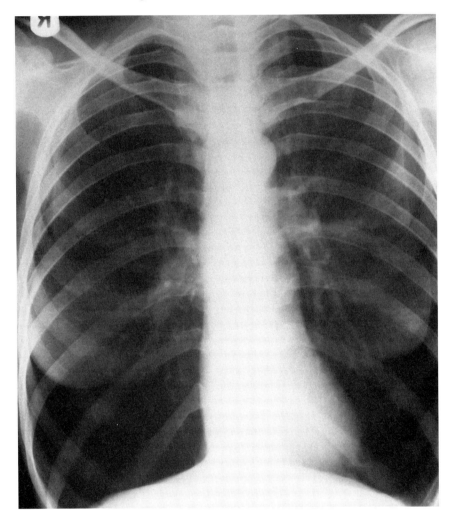

Fig. 29

Answer 29: α-1-antitrypsin (1AT) deficiency

Findings: The features of predominantly basal emphysema are present. There is flattening of the hemidiaphragms; decreased lower lobe and right upper lobe vascularity with redistribution of blood to the left upper zone. Bullae are present at the lung bases. Bilateral gynaecomastia is also present due to chronic liver disease.

1AT is a proteolytic inhibitor which is synthesized in the liver and released into the serum. 1AT deficiency has an autosomal recessive mode of inheritance with onset at 20 to 30 years of age. The absence of 1AT results in digestion of the alveolar basement membrane by elastases released by neutrophils and alveolar macrophages during episodes of bacterial infection. This results in the development of panacinar emphysema.

The clinical course is of progressively deteriorating pulmonary function. Smoking accelerates the disease process, with symptoms developing about 10 years earlier than in non-smokers. Homozygous patients may also develop hepatic cirrhosis and this patient had oesophageal varices.

CT may be used to demonstrate the disease. The predominantly basal emphysema is well shown and 40% of cases have bullae. Bronchial wall thickening is found in 40% of cases and bronchiectasis may also be seen.

Question 30

This is an axial high resolution CT (using 'lung windows') of a 68-year-old lady who kept parrots. She gave a history of several months of decreasing exercise tolerance with intermittent exacerbations. What are the CT findings? What is the most likely diagnosis?

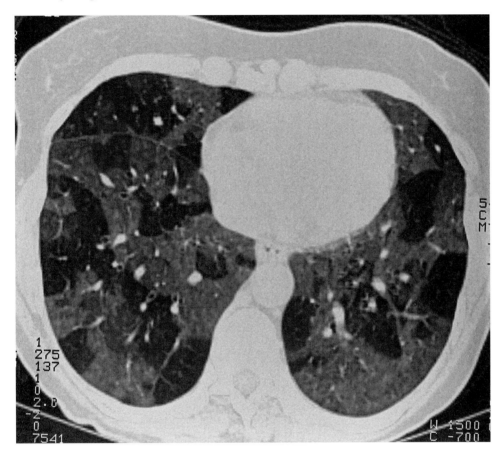

Fig. 30

Answer 30: Acute extrinsic allergic alveolitis (EAA)

Findings: A mosaic pattern of higher (light grey) and lower (black) attenuation is seen. The higher attenuation regions, also described as 'ground glass' in appearance, represent an alveolitis whilst the black areas represent patchy air trapping, a feature seen on lung function tests.

EAA results from repeated inhalation of particulate (1 to 5μm) organic antigens: Farmer's lung, Bagassosis, mushroom worker's lung, bird-fancier's lung, and malt-worker's lung are examples. The particles penetrate to the alveoli and result in an inflammatory reaction (probably combined type III and IV hypersensitivity mechanisms). There are three patterns of illness: acute, subacute, and chronic. The acute form presents 4 to 8 hours after exposure to the antigen. Examination of patients reveals crackles and, in more severe cases, tachypnoea and cyanosis. Respiratory function testing shows a mixed restrictive and obstructive pattern. The CXR may be normal in acute EAA. The most common finding in the acute and subacute phases is multiple pulmonary nodules, measuring less than 3 mm in diameter, superimposed on a background ground glass appearance. The nodules may appear within 4 hours of exposure and take weeks to months to resolve. The subacute pattern is of acute bouts on top of a progressive decline in respiratory function. The chronic CXR findings result from healing by fibrosis and include reticulonodular scarring with (predominantly upper lobe) volume loss. High resolution CT (HRCT) in the acute/ subacute phase include ground glass opacity and small centrilobular nodules. In the chronic phase the spectrum of findings includes scars through to honeycombing.

When exposure to the precipitating agent ends, the illness usually spontaneously resolves.

Question 31

This 45-year-old man presented with a 3-week history of malaise, fever, dyspnoea, and cough. The CXR (Fig. 31a) was obtained. A follow-up CXR (Fig. 31b) was taken 10 days after commencement of a drug therapy. What is the diagnosis and what treatment was administered?

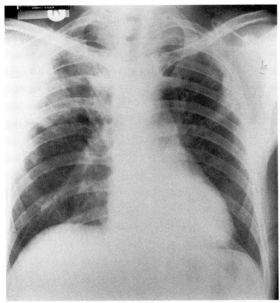

Fig. 31a

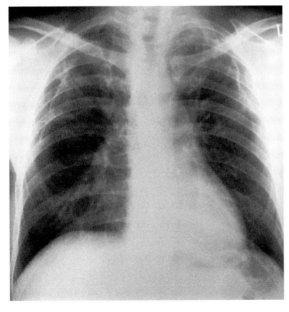

Fig. 31b

Answer 31: *Pulmonary eosinophilia treated with steroids (oral)*

Findings: Fig. 31a shows bilateral, ill-defined, peripheral consolidation in the mid and upper zones which does not conform to any lobar boundaries. This appearance has been likened to pulmonary oedema in reverse ('photographic negative'). There has been dramatic improvement on the follow-up CXR (Fig. 31b).

Pulmonary eosinophilia is defined as an eosinophilic lung infiltrate usually associated with a blood eosinophilia. Approximately a third of patients have a history of atopy. Restrictive lung function tests are found with impairment of gas exchange. The commonest cause in the United Kingdom is aspergillus but in the majority of cases the aetiology is unknown.

Causes of pulmonary eosinophilia are:

- parasites   *Ascaris lumbricoides*
                     Strongyloides stercoralis
                     Ankylostoma duodenale
                     Wuchereria bancrofti (filariasis)
                     Toxocara canis
                     Schistosoma spp.
- fungi   *Aspergillus fumigatus*
- drugs   penicillin
                     sulphonamides
                     nitrofurantoin
                     chlorpropamide
- cryptogenic (Loffler's syndrome).

Steroid therapy is rapidly effective within a few days with complete resolution of the radiographic and lung function test abnormalities. An underlying cause should be sought. Relapse may occur following cessation of therapy, requiring reinstitution.

Question 32

This 66-year-old woman presented with haemoptysis. She gave a history of TB as a young woman What abnormalities are there and how would you confirm your diagnosis?

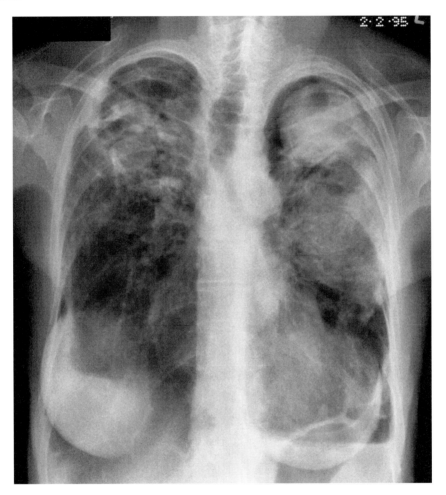

Fig. 32

Answer 32: Bilateral aspergillomas (mycetomas)

Findings: Bilateral upper zone fibrosis is present with elevation of both hila. Solid masses (aspergillomas) are seen within pulmonary cavities outlined by a rim of air in both apices.

A mycetoma is a mass of aspergillus hyphae within a cavity, usually intrapulmonary. The fungus ball may be attached to the wall of the cavity in the following: old tuberculosis, sarcoid, and ankylosing spondylitis. Fungal invasion into adjacent lung does not occur without compromised (local or general) immunity. The majority of patients are elderly males. Haemoptysis is reported in 50 to 80% of cases. Occasionally, a fungus ball may be an incidental finding. Features on examination are usually non-specific. Precipitating antibodies to aspergillus antigen are found in 90%, but are non-specific because they may also be positive in other forms of aspergillus infection. The diagnosis therefore relies on imaging. The CXR shows a soft tissue mass within a cavity: usually found in the upper lobes, or apical segment of the lower lobes. CT (Fig. 32a) more clearly demonstrates the lesion (arrows), with air spaces seen inside the aspergilloma, giving it a 'sponge-like' appearance.

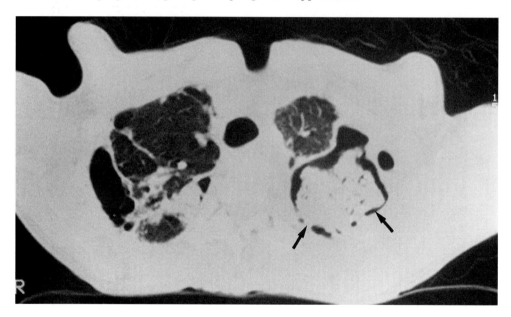

Fig. 32a   CT scan through the lung apices showing a left aspergilloma in a cavity.

Question 33

This CXR is of a 68-year-old man with a cough and progressively increasing shortness of breath. Give two abnormalities.

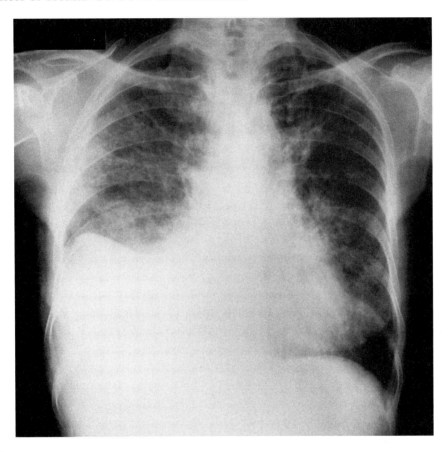

Fig. 33

Answer 33: *Right subpulmonic pleural effusion and lymphangitis carcinomatosa*

Findings: The apparent elevated right hemidiaphragm is due to subpulmonic pleural fluid. Coarse pulmonary reticular opacities are seen bilaterally, predominantly on the right. There are also Kerley B lines indicative of interstitial oedema due to malignant lymphatic infiltration and obstruction. The heart size is normal. These are the features of lymphangitis carcinomatosa (most commonly seen in bronchial, breast, and stomach cancers) with a right subpulmonic effusion.

Occasionally, pleural fluid collects inferior to the lung (subpulmonic) rather than diffusing throughout the pleural cavity. The subpulmonic fluid may accumulate unilaterally (more often on the right) or bilaterally. A large volume of fluid may accumulate in this site and be erroneously ascribed to elevation of the hemidiaphragm. The following are radiological features of a subpulmonic effusion.

1. The highest point of the pseudo-diaphragm of a subpulmonic effusion lies more lateral than that of the normal diaphragm and the medial slope is gradual and the lateral steep. These features are accentuated on expiratory films.
2. The horizontal fissure lies closer to the 'diaphragm' than usual.
3. There is usually blunting of the lateral and posterior costophrenic recesses by a small amount of fluid.
4. On the left there is increased separation of the gastric air bubble and lung.
5. There may be features related to the cause of the effusion on the CXR, for example cardiomegaly in heart failure.

Up to 300 ml can accumulate in the posterior costophrenic recess before the fluid is seen on the frontal CXR. As little as 25 ml can be seen on a lateral decubitus view.

Question 34

What does this chest radiograph demonstrate?

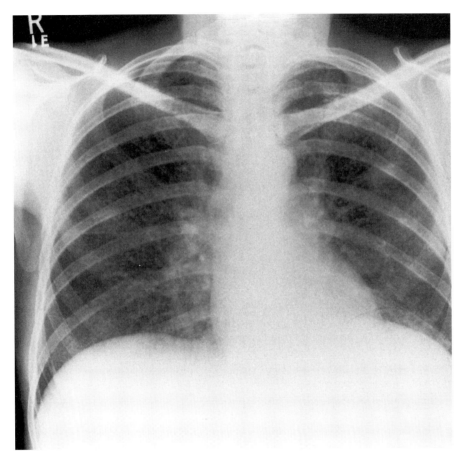

Fig. 34

Answer 34: Miliary pulmonary nodules (1 to 3 mm)

The differential diagnosis of multiple pulmonary nodules is dependent on the size of the nodules and their density:

- nodules (<2 mm)
  miliary TB
  fungi
  sarcoid
  thyroid carcinoma metastases
  lymphoma
  acute extrinsic allergic alveolitis
  pneumoconiosis/ haemosiderosis (may be dense)

- nodules/ masses (>5 mm)
  metastases
  lymphoma
  abscesses
  granulomata
  arteriovenous malformations
  infarcts
  progressive massive fibrosis.

Question 35

This 34-year-intravenous drug abuser presented with a fever and cough. What is the diagnosis?

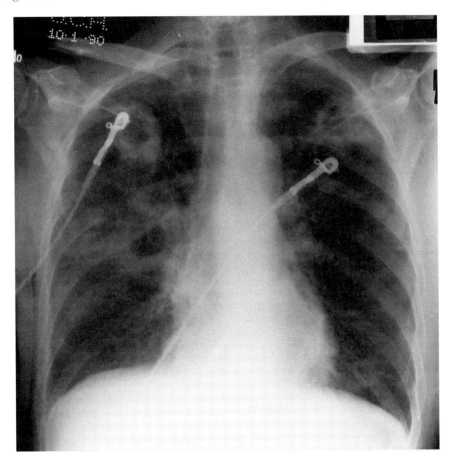

Fig. 35

Answer 35: Staphylococcal abscesses

Findings: There are multiple pulmonary cavities with fluid levels with variable surrounding parenchymal opacification.

Other causes of pulmonary cavities include:

- cavitating pneumonias (including *Staphylococcus*, *Klebsiella*, tuberculosis);
- neoplasia (carcinoma, squamous metastases);
- cavitating pulmonary infarcts;
- vasculitis (Wegener's);
- connective tissue disease (rheumatoid nodules);
- traumatic haematoma.

Predisposing factors for developing pulmonary abscesses may be: intravenous drug abuse, alcoholism, immunodeficiency, congenital heart disease, indwelling catheters, haemodialysis shunts, or cutaneous infection.

This patient is an intravenous drug abuser and the abscesses result from septic pulmonary emboli which have become lodged in the pulmonary arterial tree. The most common organisms are *Staphylococcus aureus* (as in this case) and *Streptococci*.

Question 36

This 32-year-old man presented with several months of dry cough. What is the most likely diagnosis? Describe the abnormality.

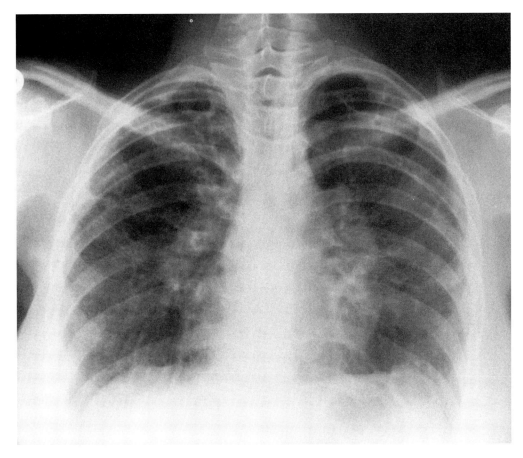

Fig. 36

Answer 36: Sarcoidosis

Findings: (1)   bilateral hilar lymphadenopathy;

                    (2)   bilateral, predominantly mid- and upper-zone reticulonodular opacities with some loss of volume;

                    (3)   apical bullae, more severe on the left.

Sarcoidosis is a multisystem disease characterized by non-caseating granulomas, most commonly involving the lungs, which either resolve (80%) or lead to the formation of fibrous tissue (20%). The CXR is abnormal in more than 90% of patients. Lymphadenopathy is the most common finding, seen in over 75%, usually with bilateral hilar and paratracheal lymph node enlargement. Pulmonary abnormality is demonstrated very rarely on the CXR prior to the development of lymphadenopathy. Lymphadenopathy usually resolves by 2 years but may contain egg shell calcification. The parenchymal pulmonary changes may be reversible. Nodules occur which commonly measure 2 to 4 mm in diameter and are characteristic of the disease. High resolution CT (HRCT) (Fig. 36a) classically demonstrates small nodules in a perilymphatic distribution, that is along the bronchovascular bundles, subpleurally (arrowheads), and along fissures (arrows). Distortion of the parenchyma and fibrosis may also be present. Air trapping on expiratory scans is well recognized. Sarcoid is predominately a mid zone process. Indications for treatment include progressive lung disease, arthropathy, hypercalcaemia, cardiac, ocular, central nervous system, and cutaneous involvement. Death is commonly pulmonary related.

The common differential diagnosis of hilar lymphadenopathy includes:

- sarcoid;
- malignancy (lymphoma, carcinomatosis);
- infection (TB, bacterial).

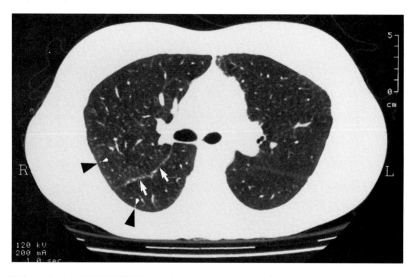

Fig. 36a   High resolution CT (HRCT) showing pulmonary sarcoidosis.

Question 37

This 24-year-old man was admitted with acute onset breathlessness and chest pain. What is the diagnosis?

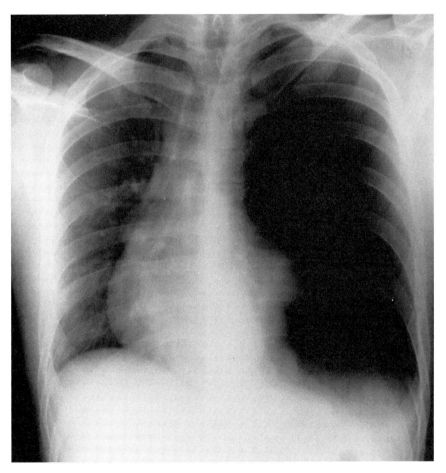

Fig. 37

Answer 37: Left tension pneumothorax

Findings: A left pneumothorax is seen associated with mediastinal shift to the right, collapse of the left lung (lobulated density inferomedially), and inversion of the left hemidiaphragm. This radiograph should not be necessary as the condition should be diagnosed clinically.

Tension pneumothorax is caused by a valvular mechanism resulting in air being sucked in during inspiration and not expelled during expiration, leading to positive intrapleural pressure. This causes mediastinal shift with compromise of venous return and cardiac output. A tension pneumothorax is a medical emergency requiring immediate insertion of a venflon and chest drain with underwater seal.

A pneumothorax may be spontaneous, traumatic, or secondary to chronic obstructive airways (COAD) disease. Secondary pneumothorax is most commonly due to airflow limitation. The decreased pulmonary reserve in this group means that a small pneumothorax may be a life- threatening event. Other causes include asthma, carcinoma, infections (e.g. *Pneumocystis carinii*), lung abscess, interstitial lung disease, and catamenial (endometriosis).

The cause of spontaneous primary pneumothorax is usually a bleb: this is seen on the acute CXR in only 15% of cases, but is identified at thoracotomy in 90%. Following a pneumothorax, the chance of a recurrence is high (40%) and the risk worsens with each subsequent event. Reabsorption of air is slow, but may be accelerated by breathing 100% oxygen. A 15% pneumothorax may take 10 days to resolve. Management may be conservative, with aspiration, chest tube drainage, or pleurodesis (with or without bleb resection).

Question 38

This 24-year-old asthmatic presented with chest pain and cough. What abnormalities are present?

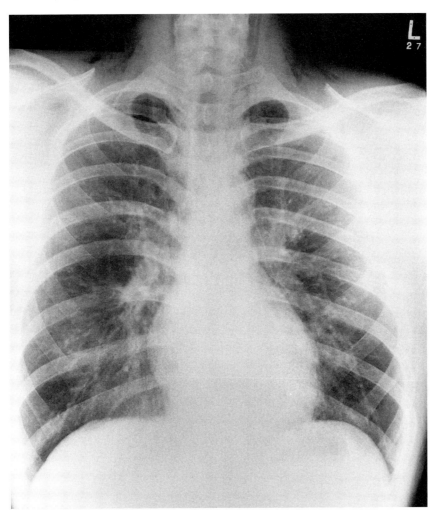

Fig. 38

Answer 38: Pneumomediastinum, surgical emphysema, and small right apical pneumothorax

A pneumomediastinum may be caused by the following:

1. Lung tear—in most cases an air leak from a small tear in the intrapulmonary airways dissects back through the lung to the hilum and into the mediastinum. The most common cause of this is asthma but any condition where there is an increase in the intra-alveolar pressure will have the same result. Thus diabetic ketoacidosis with strenuous vomiting, childbirth, artificial ventilation, pneumonias (especially those with pneumatoceles, e.g. *Pneumocystis carinii* pneumonia), chest trauma, and coughing are other causes.

2. Perforation of the oesophagus, trachea, or bronchus.

3. Perforation of an abdominal viscus with air tracking via the retroperitoneum.

A pneumomediastinum may be difficult to differentiate from a medial pneumothorax on plain films but this may be resolved with CT (Fig. 38a).

A pneumomediastinum will resorb spontaneously and usually is not of significance itself. The underlying cause must be ascertained as a major airway tear or oesophageal perforation is of great significance.

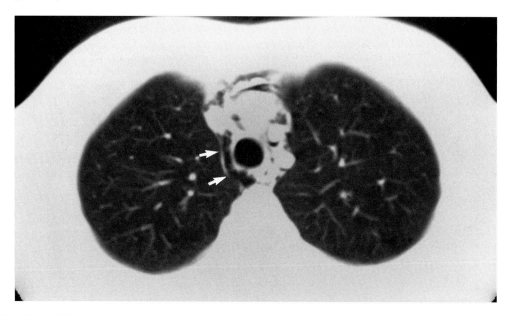

Fig. 38a   CT chest showing a pneumomediastinum (arrows).

Question 39

This 33-year-old man had a renal transplant 4 months ago. He presented with exertional dyspnoea and fever. What is the most likely diagnosis?

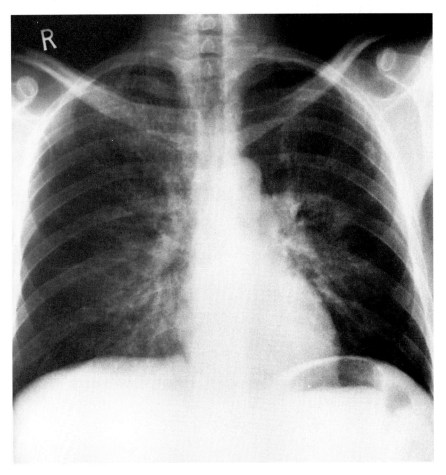

Fig. 39

Answer 39: Pneumocystis carinii pneumonia

Findings: There is bilateral perihilar parenchymal shadowing. The heart size is normal making fluid overload unlikely.

Pneumocystis carinii pneumonia is an opportunistic infection occurring in immunocompromised patients. *P. carinii* was initially classified as a protozoan but is more closely related to fungi. The chest radiograph typically shows diffuse bilateral fine reticular interstitial shadowing. Rarely nodules may be seen. A normal chest radiograph is seen in 5 to 10% at presentation. Pneumatoceles may be seen in 10% of patients with rupture resulting in a pneumothorax or pneumomediastinum. Lymphadenopathy and pleural effusions are very rare. The diagnosis is made by obtaining the organisms from induced sputum, bronchial lavage, or transbronchial biopsy. High dose trimethoprim–sulfamethoxazole is the treatment of choice with a rapid response. Resolution of chest radiographic features may lag clinical response. Fibrosis is a rare sequela. Prophylaxis with oral trimethoprim–sulfamethoxazole, nebulized pentamidine, or dapsone has dramatically reduced the incidence of this condition.

Question 40

This 50-year-old man presented with a 6-month history of increasing dyspnoea. What is the diagnosis and how would you confirm it?

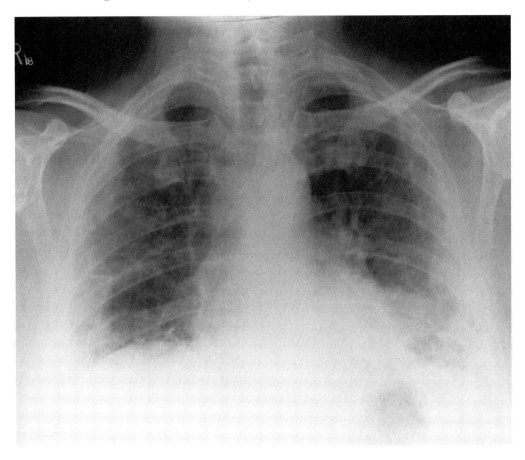

Fig. 40

Answer 40: Fibrosing alveolitis

Findings: There is bibasal interstitial shadowing with loss of lung volume (only the anterior aspect of the 5th rib can be seen, normally the 6th rib should be seen). In addition there is obscuration of the hemidiaphragms and heart borders.

Possible aetiologies are:

(1)   cryptogenic (50%);
(2)   connective tissue diseases (20%);
(3)   drugs—bleomycin, busulphan, and methotrexate;
(4)   asbestosis—usually pleural plaques and diaphragmatic calcification is present;
(5)   sarcoidosis—classically this has a mid zonal distribution but its presentation is variable.

The diagnosis may be made on high resolution CT (HRCT) (Fig. 40a) which may show ground glass shadowing, interlobular septal thickening, subpleural cyst formation (arrow), reticular fibrotic distortion (arrowheads), and traction bronchiectasis. These changes are seen in a subpleural basal distribution and are virtually diagnostic of fibrosing alveolitis. Mild lymphadenopathy is common. Different aetiologies have the same HRCT appearances. The presence of ground glass shadowing is suggestive of active alveolitis and so a potentially reversible process. The diagnosis can be confirmed by transbronchial or open lung biopsy. Treatment is with steroids with limited success. Lung transplantation is an option in appropriate candidates. There is a 50% 5-year mortality rate, death occurring from respiratory failure, pulmonary hypertension, and lung carcinoma.

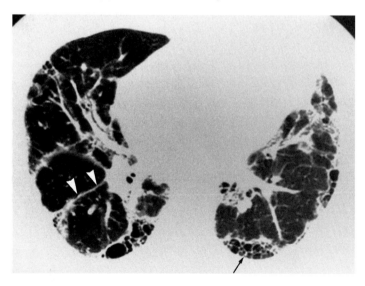

Fig. 40a   High resolution CT (HRCT) demonstrating basal pulmonary fibrosis.

Question 41

This 18-year-old man presented with recurrent pneumonias. What is the diagnosis?

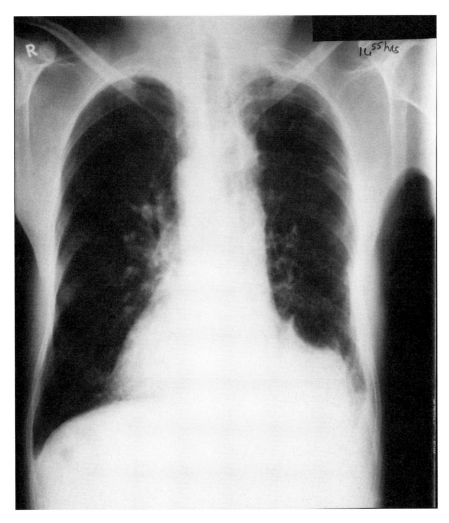

Fig. 41

Answer 41: Kartagener's syndrome with consolidation of the left lower zone (left middle and lower lobe)

Findings: There is situs inversus as evidenced by dextrocardia and the stomach bubble under the right hemidiaphragm. Consolidation of the left lower zone is present with obscuration of the heart border and left hemidiaphragm. Cystic bronchiectasis is seen adjacent to both hila and predisposes to recurrent pneumonias. A small left pleural effusion is also present.

Kartagener's syndrome is characterized by situs inversus, bronchiectasis, and chronic sinusitis, and has a strong familial tendency. It is due to mucociliary dysfunction which results in failure to clear pathogens causing bronchiectasis and sinusitis. Patients are also subfertile because of spermatic and, more rarely, fallopian tube dysmotility.

CARDIOVASCULAR SYSTEM

Question 42

This 67-year-old man presented with a 4-hour history of central chest pain radiating to the back. His electrocardiogram (ECG) was diagnostic of an acute myocardial infarction. What is the diagnosis and how would you confirm it?

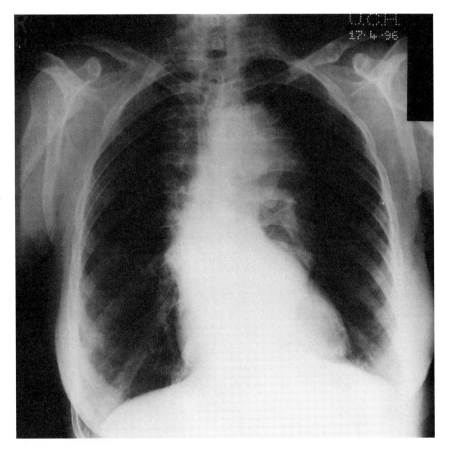

Fig. 42

Answer 42: Dissecting aortic aneurysm

Findings: The chest radiograph shows gross widening of the mediastinum and enlargement of the aortic contour. Other radiological features that may be present are tracheal and oesophageal displacement and a shift medially in the position of a calcified aortic rim by more than 6 mm from the aortic border. The cardiac silhouette may appear enlarged due to a haemopericardium or aortic regurgitation. Pleural effusion, an extrapleural apical fluid cap, and paramediastinal widening are other well recognized features. The chest radiograph may be normal. The diagnosis may be confirmed by contrast enhanced CT (Fig. 42a, arrow demonstrating a dissection of the descending aorta), MRI, aortography, or transoesophageal echocardiography.

Aortic dissection most commonly occurs secondary to hypertension but is seen in Marfan's syndrome, Ehlers–Danlos syndrome, and pregnancy. Aortic dissection may be classified into three types after DeBakey: Type I—dissection begins in the ascending aorta and extends distally beyond the ligamentum arteriosum (29 to 34%); Type II—dissection begins in the ascending aorta and ends proximal to the innominate artery (12 to 21%); and Type III—dissection begins at the ligamentum arteriosum extending down the descending aorta (50% and best prognosis).

The dissection may involve any of the vessels arising from the aorta resulting in cerebrovascular accident, myocardial infarction, aortic regurgitation, or peripheral ischaemia. DeBakey types I and II are usually managed surgically whereas type III is managed medically with antihypertensives. Mortality for untreated dissection is 30% within the first 24 hours, therefore early diagnosis is imperative.

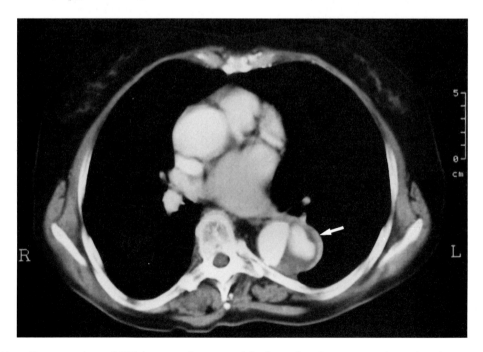

Fig. 42a   Contrast enhanced CT showing a dissection of the descending thoracic aorta (arrow) with an intimal flap seen in the centre of the vessel with contrast medium in the true and false lumens.

Question 43

What abnormality is present on the chest radiograph of this 65-year-old man? Give three complications.

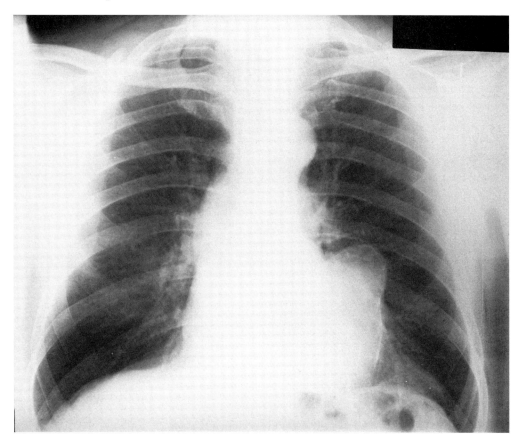

Fig. 43

Answer 43: Left ventricular aneurysm

Findings: A bulge of the left ventricular contour is seen with curvilinear calcification.
Complications include:

(1) resistant left ventricular failure;
(2) systemic embolization of associated thrombus;
(3) focus of ventricular arrhythmias;
(4) rupture.

Left ventricular aneurysm formation is a sequela of transmural myocardial infarction.
Physical examination may reveal a double apical impulse.

The electrocardiogram (ECG) shows persistent ST segment elevation. Radionuclide imaging or echocardiography are non-invasive methods of demonstrating localized paradoxical left ventricular movement during systole. Management is ventricular aneurysectomy.

Question 44

This 20-year-old man presented with hypertension. What is the diagnosis?

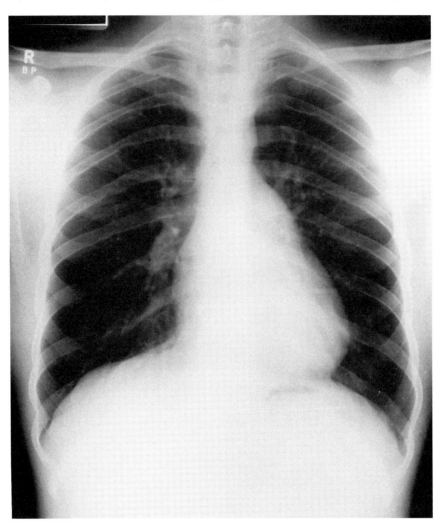

Fig. 44

Answer 44: Coarctation of the aorta

Findings: The chest radiograph shows bilateral rib notching on the inferior edge of the posterior aspects of the 3rd to 8th ribs.

Other signs that should be sought on the CXR are the 'figure 3 sign' of the aortic arch with indentation at the site of stenosis and post stenotic dilatation, and also cardiomegaly.

There are two main types of coarctation:

1. Adult type (commonest)—short discrete stenotic segment close to the ligamentum arteriosum just distal to the origin of the left subclavian artery. This type presents as an incidental finding or with hypertension. Coexistent cardiac anomalies are uncommon.
2. Infantile tubular hypoplasia—hypoplasia of a long segment of aortic arch after the origin of the innominate artery. Coexistent cardiac abnormalities are common and presentation is in the neonatal period with left ventricular failure.

Coarctation is associated with:

(1) bicuspid aortic valve;
(2) intracardiac malformations—patent ductus arteriosus, ventricular septal defect, aortic stenosis, atrial septal defect, and aortic regurgitation;
(3) Turner's syndrome;   (4)   cerebral berry aneurysms;   (5)   mycotic aneurysms distal to coarctation.

The presence of a coarctation may be confirmed by echocardiography or by magnetic resonance. Figure 44a shows a coarctation (straight arrow) distal to the origin of the left sub-clavian artery with the aortic arch (curved arrows) and descending aorta (arrowheads) labelled. Cardiac catheterization is usually only required where there are atypical signs or associated lesions. The prognosis is poor without surgery. Angioplasty may also be performed.

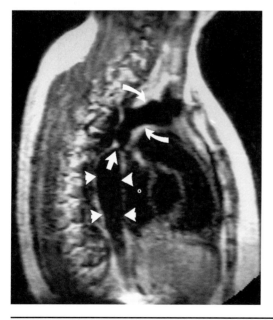

Fig. 44a   MRI section shows a coarctation of the distal aortic arch.

Question 45

This 65-year-old lady presented with chronic bilateral peripheral oedema and ascites which had failed to respond to diuretics. What abnormality is present and what is the diagnosis?

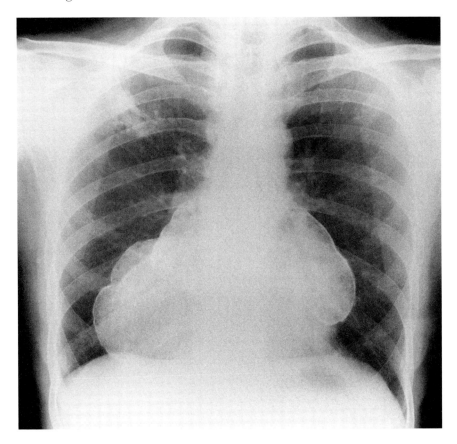

Fig. 45

Answer 45: Constrictive pericarditis associated with pericardial calcification

Findings: There is widespread curvilinear pericardial calcification with scarring in the right upper lobe indicative of previous tuberculous infection.

The commonest cause of constrictive pericarditis is idiopathic but tuberculosis was formerly the major cause. Rarer causes include postviral infection, rheumatoid arthritis, posthaemopericardium, chronic renal failure, and mediastinal radiotherapy. Constrictive pericarditis is characterized by a failure of ventricular filling and the following signs should be sought:

(1) Kussmaul's sign—an elevated jugular venous pressure (JVP) which rises instead of falling on inspiration;
(2) a prominent X and Y descent in the JVP waveform (Friedreich's sign);
(3) pulsus paradoxus—a fall of greater than 10 mmHg in systolic pressure on inspiration, the normal being 3 to 10 mmHg (i.e. an exaggeration of normal);
(4) soft heart sounds;
(5) a pericardial knock/ rub;
(6) hepatomegaly, ascites, and peripheral oedema.

The diagnosis is confirmed by echocardiography and is treated by pericardectomy.

Question 46

This 36-year-old lady had a chest X-ray performed as part of a routine insurance medical. What is the diagnosis?

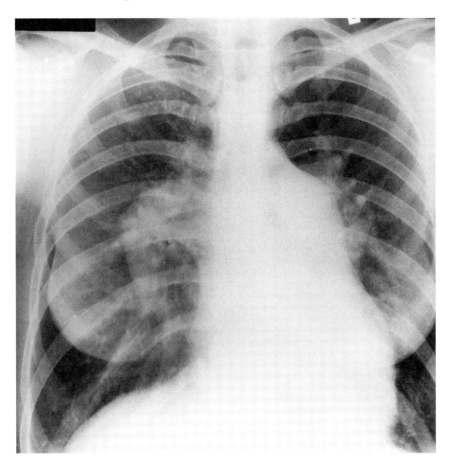

Fig. 46

Answer 46: Atrial septal defect

Findings: There is minor cardiac enlargement with rounding of the apex consistent with right ventricular enlargement/ hypertrophy. The proximal pulmonary arteries are markedly enlarged with a paucity of peripheral vascular markings (peripheral pruning) consistent with pulmonary hypertension. Calcification is seen in the main pulmonary arteries. The aortic knuckle is small.

Atrial septal defect is the second commonest congenital cardiac defect after ventricular septal defect. The condition may not be diagnosed until adulthood as there may be few symptoms and the associated murmurs may be missed. Atrial septal defect is initially an acyanotic condition characterized by left to right shunt. There is volume overload of the right ventricle resulting in pulmonary plethora (pulmonary:systemic blood flow >3:1) leading to pulmonary hypertension. Patients with an atrial septal defect develop pulmonary hypertension much later than those with ventricular septal defect, sometimes in their 40s. Once the pulmonary arterial pressure exceeds left atrial pressure the shunt will reverse and the patient becomes cyanosed. This is known as the Eisenmenger syndrome. At this point, the atrial septal defect cannot be surgically closed as the outcome would be fatal. Therefore surgical repair is the treatment of choice if the ratio of the resistance of the pulmonary to systemic system is equal to or less than 0.7.

Question 47

This 40-year-old man underwent a selective common hepatic artery angiogram for investigation of upper gastrointestinal bleeding. What is the diagnosis?

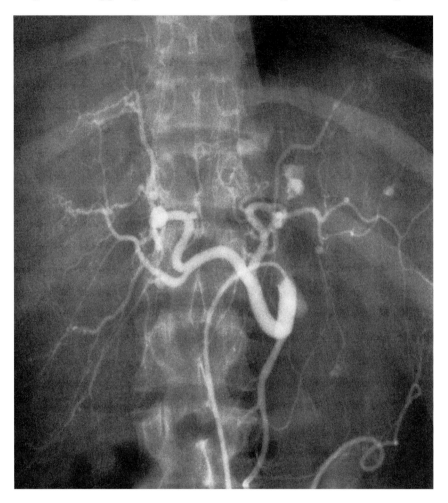

Fig. 47

Answer 47: *Polyarteritis nodosa (PAN)*

Findings: Multiple aneurysms are present on the branches of the right and left hepatic arteries.

Another possible explanation is multiple mycotic aneurysms associated with endocarditis or salmonella septicaemia and occasionally in systemic lupus erythematosus (SLE).

PAN is characterized by a vasculitis affecting the medium sized arteries with necrotizing granulomas. This process may produce aneurysms, stenoses, and occlusions. The kidney is the most commonly affected (85%) which may lead to hypertension, renal failure, infarction, or haematuria. The chest is involved in 70% with cardiac enlargement, pericardial effusion, pleural effusion, pulmonary oedema, cavitation, and haemorrhage. Involvement of the mesenteric vessels (50%) may result in abdominal pain, ulceration, gastrointestinal haemorrhage, or intestinal infarction. Cutaneous manifestations (20%) include necrotizing vasculitis, livedo reticularis, and tender subcutaneous nodules.

The condition is associated with positive hepatitis B antigenaemia, raised erythrocyte sedimentation rate (ESR), pyrexia of unknown origin, myalgia, and arthalgias. Treatment is with steroids and there is a 50% 5-year survival.

Question 48

This 26-year-old Japanese lady presented with a cerebrovascular accident. The arch aortogram is shown. What is the diagnosis?

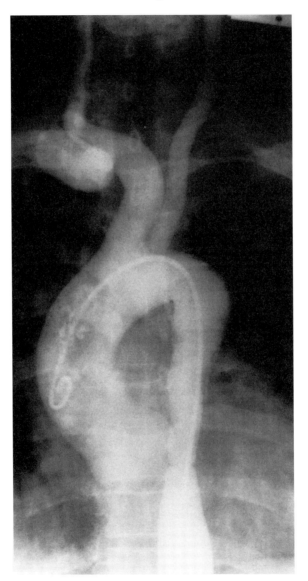

Fig. 48

Answer 48: *Takayasu's arteritis*

Findings: The left subclavian and vertebral arteries are absent . There is a fusiform aneurysm of the right subclavian and innominate arteries. There is also a stenosis in the mid descending aorta with aortic calcification.

Takayasu's arteritis (pulseless disease) occurs in young Japanese females (M:F 1:8) and is a chronic inflammatory panarteritis of unknown aetiology affecting segments of the aorta, its main branches, and pulmonary arteries. It is characterized by a prepulseless phase of a few months with fevers, weight loss, arthalgia, and myalgia followed by a pulseless phase with limb ischaemia and renovascular hypertension. The erythrocyte sedimentation rate (ESR) is elevated. The most commonly involved vessels are the left subclavian, left common carotid, innominate, and renal arteries. Angiography typically shows stenoses of varying lengths of the aorta and segmental irregular stenoses/ occlusion of major branches of the aorta near their origins. Stenotic lesions of the thoracic aorta are commoner than the abdominal aorta. Fusiform aortic aneurysms occur in 10 to 15% of cases. Frequent skip areas also are a feature. It is the only form of aortitis that produces both stenosis and occlusion. Treatment consists of steroids and angioplasty of stenotic lesions after resolution of active inflammation.

Question 49

This 76-year-old lady presented with a history of progressive dyspnoea. What is the diagnosis?

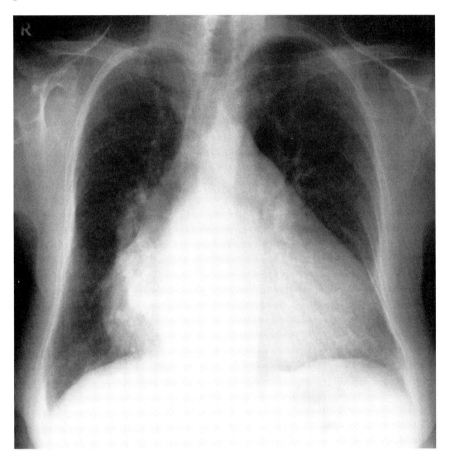

Fig. 49

Answer 49: Mixed mitral valve disease

Findings: There is cardiomegaly. Left atrial enlargement is present as evidenced by the double contour to the right heart border, prominent left atrial appendage on the left heart border, and splaying of the carina. Small pleural effusions and upper lobe venous diversion are present.

The commonest cause of this valvular disorder is rheumatic fever, although only half the patients have a positive history. Presenting features may be dyspnoea due to pulmonary venous hypertension causing pulmonary oedema, haemoptysis, systemic emboli from left atrial thrombus, palpitations secondary to atrial fibrillation, infective endocarditis, and dysphagia due to left atrial oesophageal compression. The diagnosis is confirmed by echocardiography and cardiac catheterization. Severe mitral stenosis is present when the valvular area is less than 1 cm^2.

Management is divided into medical and surgical. Medical management consists of digoxin to slow the ventricular rate in atrial fibrillation, diuretics to reduce pulmonary venous congestion, and anticoagulants especially in systemic/ pulmonary embolism and when atrial fibrillation occurs. Surgical options include valvotomy, valvuloplasty, or valve replacement.

Question 50

What is the diagnosis? Give three causes.

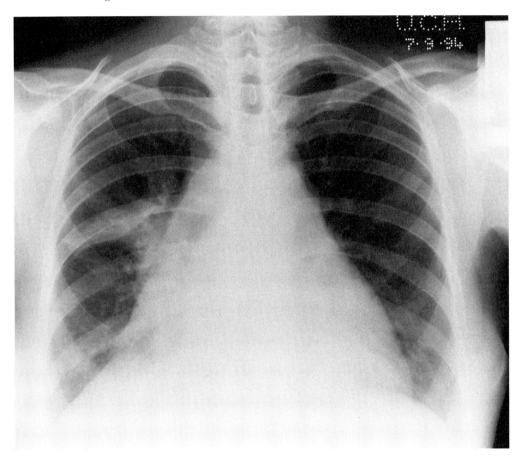

Fig. 50

Answer 50: Pericardial effusion

Findings: There is a globular-shaped, enlarged cardiac silhouette with loculated fluid in the right horizontal fissure. The diagnosis in this patient was tuberculosis. An axial CT section at the level of the pulmonary artery (Fig. 50a) in another case shows a pericardial effusion (straight arrow), right pleural effusion (curved arrow), and a right hilar bronchial carcinoma (arrowhead).

Causes of pericardial effusion are:
1. Exudate: infections—viral, pyogenic, tuberculous;
            uraemia;
            collagen vascular diseases—SLE, rheumatoid arthritis;
            neoplasm—metastases, lymphoma, mesothelioma, sarcoma.
2. Blood: trauma;
            rupture of aortic aneurysm.
3. Lymph: cardiothoracic surgery;
            obstruction of thoracic duct.
4. Transudate: congestive heart failure, hypoalbuminaemia.

The commonest causes are infective, traumatic, collagen vascular disease, uraemia, and neoplasia.

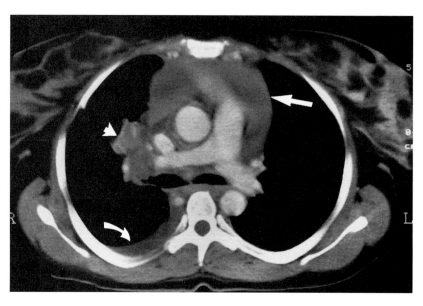

Fig. 50a   Contrast enhanced CT showing pericardial and pleural effusions secondary to a right bronchogenic carcinoma.

GASTROENTEROLOGY

Question 51

A 65-year-old man presented to casualty with a 2-hour history of left sided chest pain associated with nausea and vomiting. His serum amylase and electro-cardiogram were normal. What is the diagnosis?

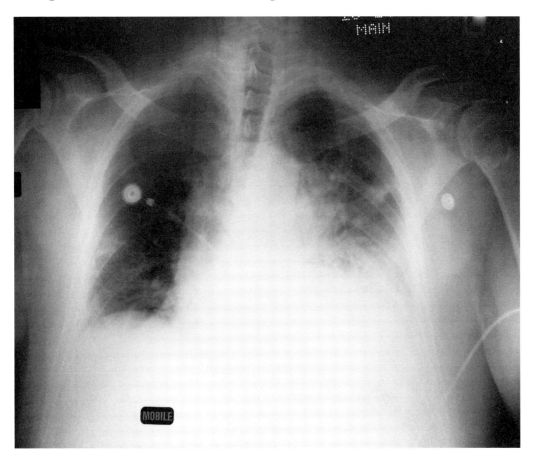

Fig. 51

Answer 51: Boerhaave's syndrome (spontaneous oesophageal rupture)

Findings: The chest radiograph shows a left pleural effusion, a pneumomediastinum (air outlining the aortic arch), and surgical emphysema on the right side of the neck.

Other radiological features which should be sought are pneumothorax, hydropneumothorax, and free subdiaphragmatic gas in distal oesophageal tears.

Boerhaave's syndrome is typically caused by forceful vomiting associated with a large intake of alcohol and/or food. Perforation most often occurs in the distal left oesophagus and is diagnosed by an oesophagogram (Fig. 51a) using water soluble contrast media. Barium is not used because of the risk of mediastinitis. Boerhaave's syndrome should be differentiated from the Mallory–Weiss syndrome in which the tear is superficial and limited to the mucosa. Boerhaave's syndrome has a high mortality as a result of shock, mediastinitis, and sepsis.

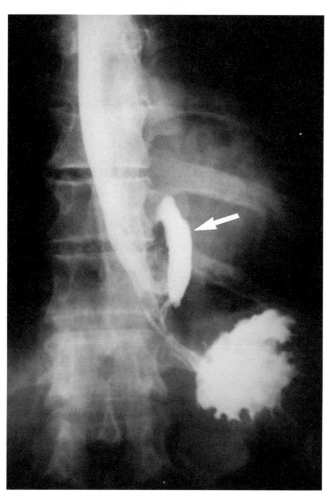

Fig. 51a   Contrast swallow demonstrating an oesophageal tear (arrow).

Question 52

What is the diagnosis and give two complications?

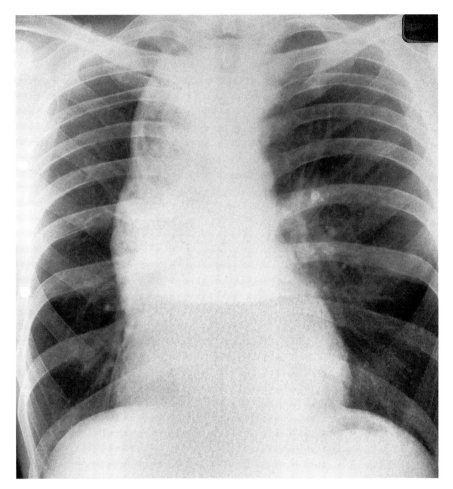

Fig. 52

Answer 52: Achalasia

Complications are aspiration and carcinoma of the oesophagus.

Findings: The chest radiograph shows a massively dilated oesophagus full of food residue. This can be confirmed by barium swallow (Fig. 52a).

The condition is characterized by failure of relaxation of the lower oesophageal sphincter resulting in proximal dilatation and there is also loss of peristaltic contractions. A decrease in the number of ganglionic cells is seen in the nerve plexus of the oesophageal wall. Chagas' disease produces a similar clinical picture. Patients usually have dysphagia for both solids and liquids and pain may be a prominent feature. The diagnosis is made by barium swallow and manometry.

The barium swallow shows oesophageal dilatation. No primary peristaltic waves pass beyond the upper thoracic oesophagus. Contrast studies classically show a 'bird-beak' appearance of the distal oesophagus with small quantities of contrast intermittently squirting into the stomach. Achalasia must be differentiated from scleroderma and a distal oesophageal carcinoma. In scleroderma, the oesophagus is usually less dilated and free gastro-oesophageal reflux is present which may result in benign peptic oesophageal stricture mimicking achalasia. Less dilatation is present with an oesophageal carcinoma. Oesophagoscopy should be performed to exclude a secondary malignancy. Treatment is via balloon dilatation or surgical intervention (myotomy).

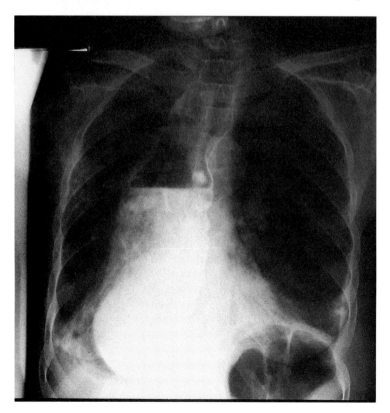

Fig. 52a Barium swallow (of another patient) showing a dilated, tortuous oesophagus containing food residue and an air–fluid level.

Question 53

This 75-year-old lady complained of dysphagia. What abnormality is present on this barium swallow and what is its significance?

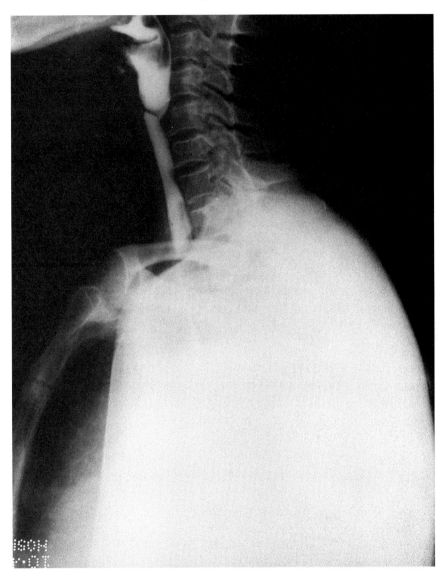

Fig. 53

Answer 53: Postcricoid oesophageal web

Findings: A web is present arising from the anterior wall of the oesophagus. It is best demonstrated on a barium distended oesophagus.

Webs are classically found in middle-aged females and consist of a thin membrane of less than 3 mm in thickness. Atrophy of the squamous epithelium in the postcricoid region occurs, near the upper oesophageal sphincter, with formation of the web. The web may be asymptomatic; produce dysphagia; or may be associated with the Plummer–Vinson syndrome (Paterson–Brown–Kelly syndrome) in which iron deficiency anaemia, glossitis, and angular stomatitis are found. Rarely dilatation is necessary to treat dysphagia. It was thought that the condition was premalignant but this association is uncertain. The web is often missed at oesophagoscopy.

Question 54

What is the diagnosis and what complications may occur?

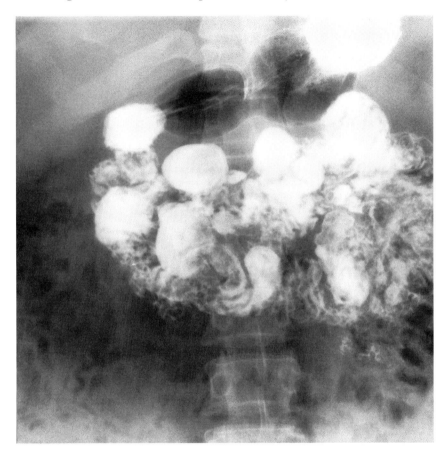

Fig. 54

Answer 54: Jejunal diverticulosis

Findings: Multiple barium-filled diverticulae are seen arising from the duodenum and jejunum.

Jejunal diverticulae are due to mucosal herniation through the submucosa and muscularis on the mesenteric border of the intestine at the entry points of blood vessels in the same manner as colonic diverticulae. Bacterial overgrowth resulting in vitamins B_{12} and K deficiency along with deconjugation of bile salts causes fat malabsorption which manifests as steatorrhoea. The condition is usually seen in elderly patients and may be complicated by perforation, diverticulitis, haemorrhage, intussusception, or intestinal obstruction. Treatment is with antibiotics to eradicate the bacterial overgrowth or resection of the diseased segment if it is localized.

Question 55

This 26-year-old patient presented with a 10-day history of bloody diarrhoea and increasing abdominal pain. What is the diagnosis and list three causes?

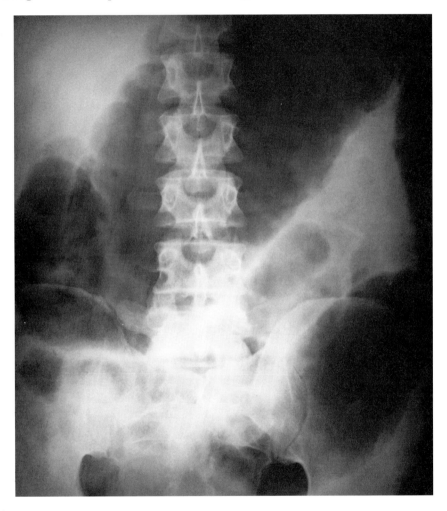

Fig. 55

Answer 55: Toxic megacolon

The causes are ulcerative colitis, Crohn's disease, pseudomembranous colitis, ischaemia, bacillary dysentery, amoebiasis, typhoid fever, cholera, and Behçet's syndrome

Findings: There is dilatation of the transverse colon with abnormal thickening of the bowel wall caused by mucosal oedema. Mucosal islands (pseudopolyps) are identified which are areas of normal mucosa. The maximum transverse colonic diameter is 12 cm (upper limit of normal is 5.5 cm). No intramural or free intraperitoneal air is seen.

Toxic megacolon is due to transmural inflammation with neuromuscular degeneration. It is important to differentiate toxic megacolon from other causes of a dilated colon where the mucosal pattern will be normal, for example ileus, pseudo obstruction, and true obstruction. As well as the radiological findings the diagnosis is also based on the patient's clinical condition, that is the presence of pyrexia, tachycardia, and leucocytosis. Perforation and ensuing peritonitis is common with a high mortality (>20%). Perforation may be heralded by air within the bowel wall. Sigmoidoscopy and rectal biopsy usually yield the underlying cause but a barium enema is contraindicated.

Fig. 55

Question 56

This 32-year-old lady complained of altered bowel habit. What abnormality is present on the barium enema (sigmoid colon view) and what is the most likely diagnosis?

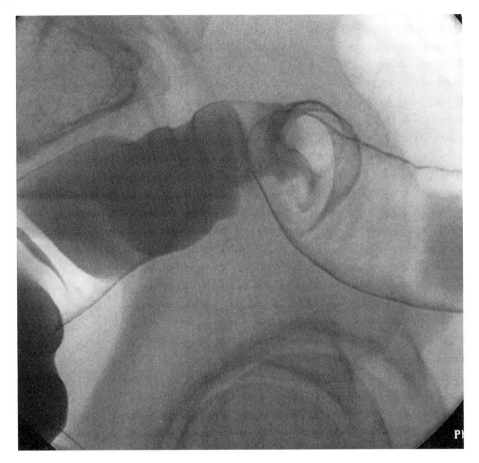

Fig. 56

Answer 56: Extrinsic lesion indenting the sigmoid colon secondary to endometriosis

Findings: An irregular stenosing lesion is seen in the sigmoid colon with a smooth but crenated mucosal fold pattern indicating that it is extra mural adherent to the serosal surface

The differential diagnosis includes: metastatic deposits from carcinoma of the ovary, colon, or stomach; radiotherapy; and pelvic inflammatory disease. Endometriosis is the condition where functional endometrial epithelium is found outside the uterine cavity. It occurs in the third and fourth decades and is associated with infertility. Endometriotic deposits involve the bowel in 12 to 20% of cases; most commonly the rectosigmoid colon. They are described as having the appearance of chocolate cysts at laparoscopy because they contain old, altered blood. They may cause change in bowel habit, rectal bleeding, and pain. Symptoms are exacerbated during menstruation.

Question 57

This barium enema was performed on a 26-year-old man with altered bowel habit. What is the diagnosis?

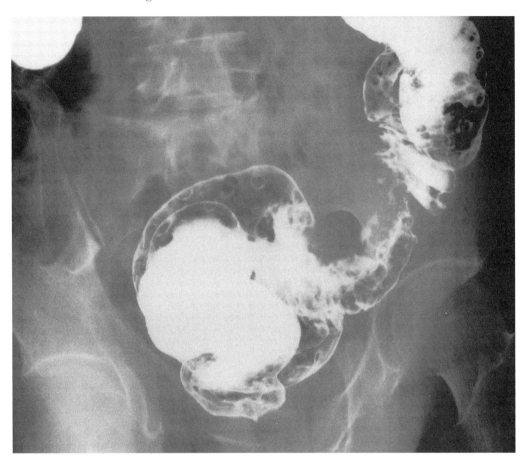

Fig. 57

Answer 57: Cancer of the descending colon complicating familial polyposis coli

Findings: Multiple small polyps (halo-like lesions) are seen in the sigmoid and distal descending colon. There is an annular stenosing carcinoma in the descending colon, with irregularity and destruction of the mucosal folds.

Familial adenomatous polyposis coli is an autosomal dominant disease with 80% penetration. The condition occurs sporadically in one-third. Polyps appear around the 2nd or 3rd decade of life, causing rectal bleeding, diarrhoea, and mucus discharge.

The colon is affected in all patients with development of carcinoma at a rate of 30% after 10 years and 100% after 20 years. There is a high proportion (80%) of multifocal carcinomas. Therefore a prophylactic proctocolectomy is performed once the condition is diagnosed. Relatives should be screened by colonoscopy from their early teens to middle age.

The condition is also associated with hamartomas of the stomach (50%), adenomas of the duodenum (25%), and periampullary carcinoma.

Gardner's syndrome is a variant of this condition. In addition to the colonic adenomas, skull osteomata, epidermoid cysts with desmoid tumour formation, and dental abnormalities are found.

Question 58

This 65-year-old patient complained of non-specific abdominal pain. What is the diagnosis?

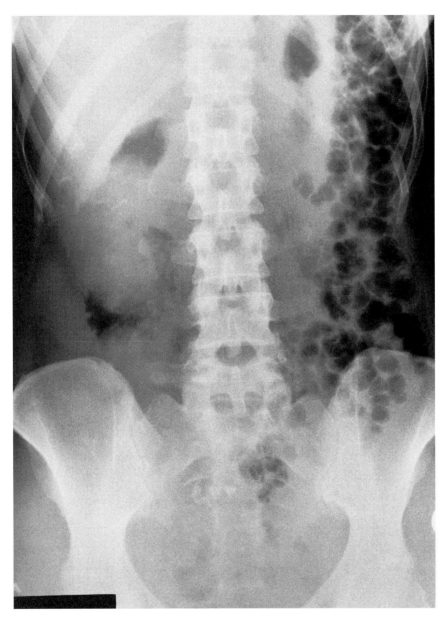

Fig. 58

Answer 58: Pneumatosis coli

Findings: There are widespread, gas-filled cysts seen along the contour of the colonic wall. The diagnosis can be confirmed on barium enema (Fig. 58a, from a different patient).

In pneumatosis coli (pneumatosis cystoides intestinalis), nitrogen cysts occur in the sub-mucosal and subserosal layers of the bowel wall. They are usually on the mesenteric side of the bowel. They may rupture resulting in pneumoperitoneum without peritonitis. Recognition of pneumatosis coli as the underlying cause is essential to avoid unnecessary laparatomy.

The commonest causes are chronic obstructive airways disease, asthma, connective tissue diseases (scleroderma, polymyositis), and, rarely, inflammatory bowel disease. Pneumatosis coli is commonest in the sigmoid and descending colon.

Patients are usually asymptomatic but may present with vague abdominal pain, diarrhoea, or constipation. Treatment is not necessary but if the patient is symptomatic hyperbaric oxygen therapy may be used. Since the gas in the cyst is predominantly nitrogen, oxygen therapy lowers the partial pressure of other gases in the blood so facilitating diffusion of nitrogen from the cysts. In contrast to pneumatosis coli, the presence of linear intramural gas is a sign of bowel necrosis/ infarction.

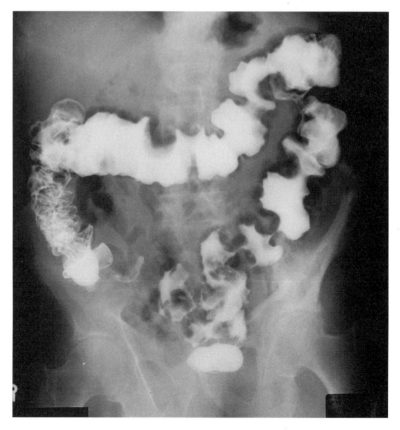

Fig. 58a   Barium enema showing pneumatosis coli.

Question 59

What abnormality is present on this barium swallow?

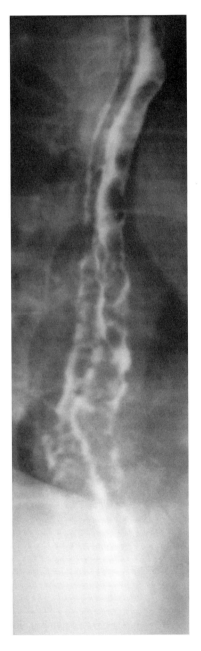

Fig. 59

Answer 59: Oesophageal varices

Findings: There are multiple serpiginous filling defects interrupting the normal mucosal folds of the oesophagus.

Oesophageal varices result from portal venous hypertension which induces large collateral channels at the portosystemic anastomotic channels. The main sites of portosystemic anastomoses are the gastro-oesophageal junction, rectum (causing haemorrhoids), left renal vein, lumbar veins, falciform ligament of the liver, and veins of the anterior abdominal wall (known as a caput medusae).

The causes of portal hypertension may be subdivided into:

(1)   extrahepatic—portal vein thrombosis;
(2)   intrahepatic—cirrhosis (commonest cause);
(3)   posthepatic—Budd–Chiari syndrome, constrictive pericarditis, veno-occlusive disease, and right heart failure.

Oesophageal varices resulting from portal hypertension occur in the distal oesophagus and are known as 'uphill varices' since blood flows from the portal vein via the azygos vein into the superior vena cava (SVC). Varices may occur in the upper third of the oesophagus and are known as 'downhill varices' since blood flows from the SVC via the azygos vein into the inferior vena cava/ portal vein. This type are rare and occur as a result of SVC obstruction distal to the entry site of the azygos vein as a result of lung cancer, lymphoma, retrosternal goitre, thymoma, or mediastinal fibrosis.

Variceal bleeding occurs in 28% within 3 years and has a high mortality. It constitutes a medical emergency. A recent radiological intervention is transjugular intrahepatic porto-systemic shunting (TIPPS) which reduces portal pressure and decreases mortality but has an increased risk of encephalopathy.

Question 60

This 26-year-old renal transplant patient complained of dysphagia. What is the diagnosis?

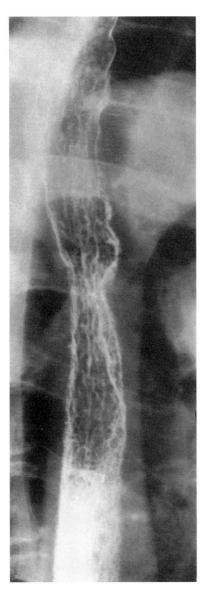

Fig. 60

Answer 60: Oesophageal candidiasis

Findings: The barium swallow shows mucosal ulceration and longitudinal plaques made up of tiny nodules.

Predisposing factors to oesophageal candidiasis include immunocompromised patients (haematologic disease, leukaemia, diabetes mellitus, steroids, chemotherapy, radiotherapy, HIV), antibiotic therapy, scleroderma, oesophageal strictures, and achalasia. Candidiasis is the commonest fungal opportunistic infection. There is a predilection for the lower half of the oesophagus but the whole oesophagus is frequently involved. Herpes simplex and cytomegalovirus (CMV) oesophagitis may be indistinguishable but herpes simplex tends to give superficial punctate ulceration on a background of normal mucosa. CMV infection is associated with severe odynophagia with larger ulcers near the gastro-oesophageal junction. Oesophageal candidiasis responds well to systemic antifungal therapy.

Question 61

This superior mesenteric artery (SMA) angiogram was performed on a 75-year-old lady with profuse rectal bleeding. What is the most likely diagnosis?

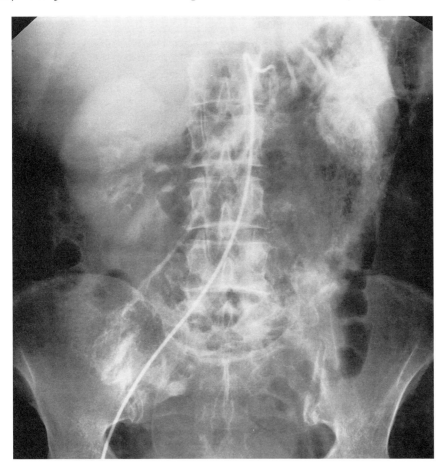

Fig. 61

Answer 61: Caecal angiodysplasia

Findings: A catheter is present in the origin of the SMA. The capillary phase of the injection is shown. A vascular blush is seen in the region of the caecum indicative of an angiodysplasia. Early venous filling is another feature (seen to the right of the catheter).

Colonic angiodysplasia predominantly affects the middle aged and elderly. The incidence is 2% at autopsy. Aortic stenosis is associated in 20%. Angiodysplasia consists of vascular ectasias with the majority occurring in the caecum and ascending colon. The descending and sigmoid colon is affected in 25% of cases. Patients may present with acute or chronic blood loss. The lesions are multiple in 20% and demonstration of an angiodysplastic lesion does not prove that it is the source of haemorrhage. Occasionally, contrast extravasation may be seen indicating ulceration and focal bleeding. Active bleeding of at least 30 ml/hour is needed to demonstrate a bleeding point angiographically. Active bleeding may also be demonstrated using radionuclide studies with EDTA^{51Cr} or Tc^{99m} labelled red blood cells. Management is surgical although at operation the surgeon may have to perform a blind resection as the lesion cannot be palpated or visualized. At angiography the feeding arterial supply can be marked by lodging a wire in it which can be palpated at operation thus aiding the surgeon in resection of the occult angiodysplasia. The pathologist usually cannot locate the lesion without special localization techniques.

Question 62

This 56-year-lady was admitted with acute abdominal pain. A supine abdominal radiograph was obtained. What abnormalities are present?

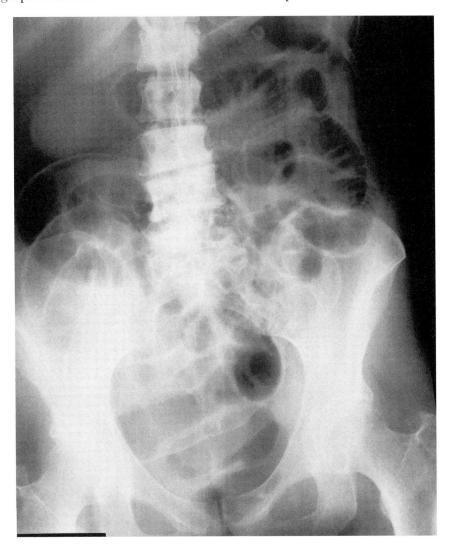

Fig. 62

Answer 62: Free intraperitoneal air (pneumoperitoneum) secondary to a perforated viscus

Findings: Both sides of bowel wall can be seen which is a feature of free intraperitoneal air known as Rigler's sign. This is best seen in the left upper quadrant. In addition, air outlines the gallbladder in the right upper quadrant. Approximately 50% of patients with free intraperitoneal gas will have a collection of air adjacent to the liver lying in the subhepatic space and hepatorenal space (Morrison's pouch) on a supine film.

Other signs of free intraperitoneal gas are:

(1)   air outlining the falciform ligament of the liver;
(2)   air outlining the umbilical ligaments;
(3)   air interposed between the colon and properitoneal fat stripe of the abdominal wall;
(4)   a central collection of gas anterior to loops of bowel;
(5)   on an erect chest radiograph air collects under the hemidiaphragms (Fig. 62a).

A left lateral decubitus film (patient lying on their left side) detects as little as 1 ml of free air. The patient remains in position for 5 to 10 min prior to taking the radiograph to allow any air to rise. However, it is important to recognize the signs of free intraperitoneal gas on supine films as the patient may be too ill to obtain other films.

Certain conditions may mimic pneumoperitoneum:

(1)   Chilaiditi's syndrome (bowel between liver and diaphragm);
(2)   cysts in pneumatosis coli;   (3)   subphrenic abscess;
(4)   subdiaphragmatic fat;   (5)   uneven diaphragm;
(6)   subpulmonic pneumothorax;   (7)   curvilinear basal lung collapse.

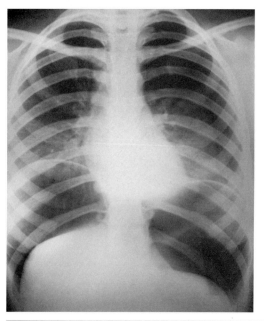

Fig. 62a   A large amount of free intraperitoneal air seen on an erect chest radiograph.

Question 63

What abnormalities are present on this barium enema and what is the underlying disease?

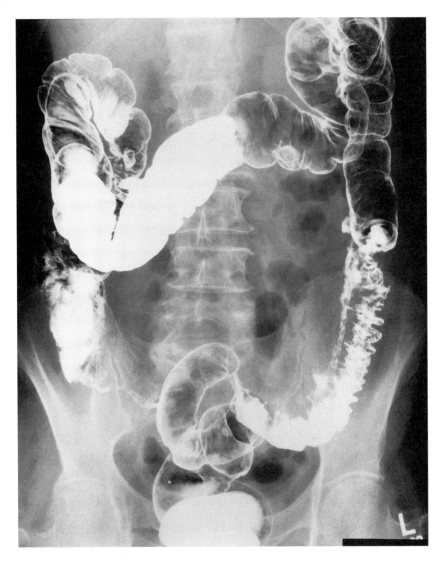

Fig. 63

Answer 63: Crohn's disease

Findings: A colo–colic fistula is seen adjacent to the descending colon. The mucosal pattern is abnormal with deep (rose thorn) ulcers which the fistula joins. There is also abnormal mucosal coating in the hepatic and splenic flexures consistent with early aphthous ulceration (barium in a central ulcer surrounded by a translucent halo of oedematous mucosa). In the sigmoid colon there is a stricture.

Crohn's disease is an inflammatory bowel disease which may affect any part of the intestine but most commonly affects the terminal ileum. The colon is involved in approximately a third of patients. Crohn's disease is characterized by transmural inflammation with asymmetric bowel wall involvement and skip lesions. The earliest radiographic change is aphthous ulceration which occurs in the mucosal lymphoid tissue. With disease progression, the following may be seen on barium studies:

(1) deep ulceration known as rose thorn ulcers;
(2) cobblestone appearance due to longitudinal and transverse ulcers separated by areas of oedema;
(3) strictures which may be inflammatory or fibrotic;
(4) pseudosacculation—bulging area of normal wall opposite affected scarred wall (seen in descending colon adjacent to the fistula in this case);
(5) bowel wall thickening secondary to inflammation.

HEPATOBILIARY DISEASE

Question 64

This 76-year-old lady presented with a 5-day history of increasing abdominal pain and distension with vomiting. What abnormality has been arrowed on this plain abdominal film? Give two further abnormalities. What is the diagnosis?

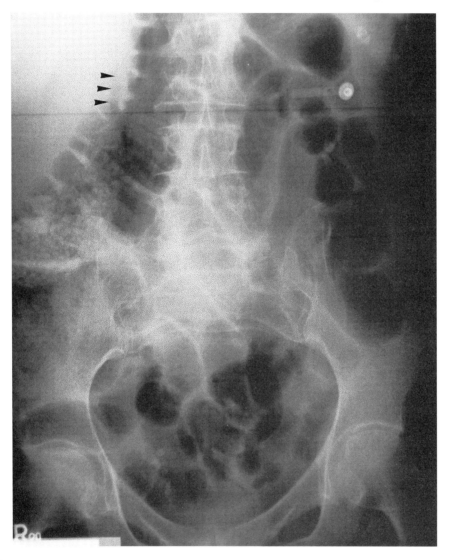

Fig. 64

Answer 64: Gallstone ileus

Abnormalities are (1) aerobilia (air in the biliary tree arrowed) seen over the right upper quadrant; (2) small bowel obstruction; (3) multiple radio-opaque gallstones in the gallbladder.

Findings: A branching lucency (air) is seen over-lying the liver. In addition, there are loops of dilated, gas-containing small bowel due to the small intestinal obstruction resulting from the impaction of the calculus at the ileocaecal valve.

Hepatic linear or branching lucencies may result from air in the biliary tree or portal venous system. The former is often located close to the hepatic hilum and is in continuity with air in the common bile duct and duodenum. Air in the biliary tree may be due to: post-ERCP or surgery, biliary calculi, emphysematous cholecystitis, and malignant fistula formation. When due to biliary calculi, the stone may have passed through the biliary tree and resulted in a patulous ampulla of Vater, or (rarely) eroded through the gallbladder wall into adjacent bowel. Any surgery resulting in bypass, or dysfunction of the biliary ampulla, may result in aerobilia. Air in the portal veins lies peripherally within the liver, where it has embolized in a distal part of the venous system. In this case, a large, solitary biliary calculus has eroded into the duodenum and then passed down the small intestine to become impacted at the ileocaecal valve (site of impaction in 75%). This has resulted in aerobilia, through the passage of gas from the duodenum into the gallbladder and the biliary ducts, and small intestinal obstruction. Surgical relief of the obstruction was required. Gallstone ileus results in 1 to 3% of intestinal obstructions (up to 20% above the age of 70) and has a high mortality. The commonest age range is 65 to 75 years (M:F 1:7). Less than 1% of patients with cholelithiasis develop gallstone ileus and only 15% of patients with gallbladder perforation by a calculus go on to intestinal obstruction.

Question 65

This is a hepatic ultrasound on a 43-year-old male who presented with a 10-day history of fever, vomiting, and upper abdominal pain. What has been measured?

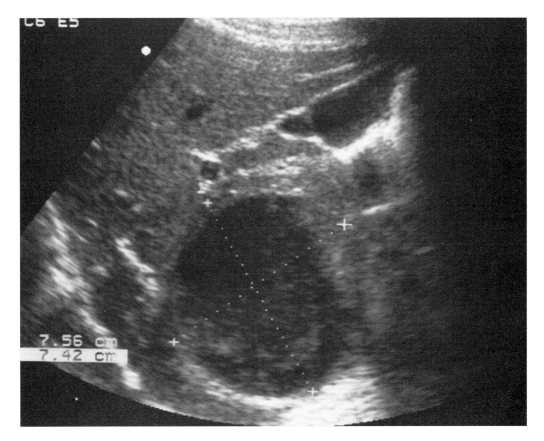

Fig. 65

Answer 65: Pyogenic liver abscess

Findings: Within the liver there is a rounded area of decreased echogenicity (darker than the rest of the liver).

Pyogenic liver abscesses are uncommon, occurring most frequent in the 40 to 60 year age group. The underlying cause may be: ascending cholangitis (commonest cause with multiple abscesses found in over 90%); portal phlebitis (secondary to an infective focus within the drainage area of the portal vein); pyogenic hepatic arterial emboli; extension from an adjacent septic process; and traumatic introduction of septic material. Abscess formation from appendicitis and diverticulitis is now rare. In adults, the most common organism isolated is *Streptococcus milleri* and in children it is *Staphylococcus aureus*. The clinical presentation of an hepatic abscess is non-specific resulting in a high mortality (>70%) prior to the introduction of cross-sectional imaging. Patients present with: pyrexia, abdominal pain, vomiting, night sweats, and jaundice.

CT (Fig. 65a) is the investigation of choice, with a sensitivity of over 95%. The abscess is usually shown as a rounded, well-defined, hypodense lesion with a peripheral rim that enhances after the administration of contrast. In some cases, septation or a cluster of cavities is seen. Ultrasound features are variable, but scanning of a liquefied abscess commonly shows a well-defined hypoechoic lesion with a mildly hyperechoic rim and distal enhancement. There may be debris within the abscess and strongly echogenic foci resulting from gas are seen in 20% of cases. The sensitivity for lesions varies with size, but is up to 90% for 15 mm diameter abscesses.

Treatment is with drainage, where possible via an image-guided, percutaneous route and antibiotics (with sensitivities confirmed by the results of culture from the abscess). Therapy should also be aimed at the underlying cause of the abscess.

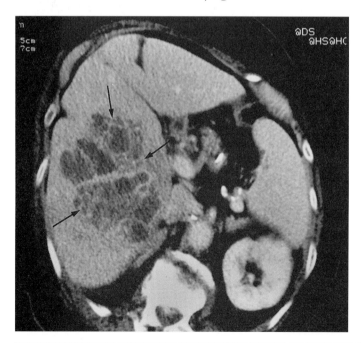

Fig. 65a Hepatic abscess. An enhanced CT section showing a rim enhancing, multiloculated area of low density in the right lobe of liver (arrows).

Question 66

This is an axial enhanced CT section through the upper abdomen of a New Zealander. What is the most likely diagnosis?

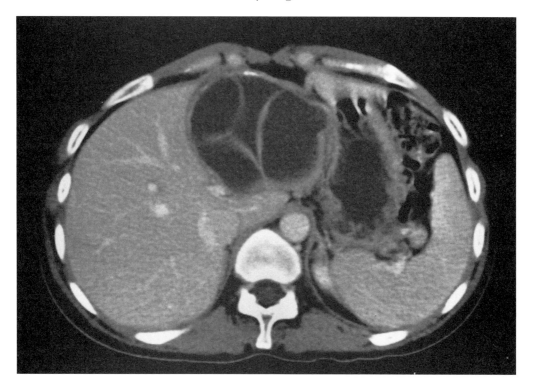

Fig. 66

Answer 66: Hydatid cyst

Findings: A multiseptated encapsulated cyst is seen in the left lobe of the liver.

Hydatid cysts result from infection by *Echinococcus granulosus*. Man is an accidental host. The definitive host is the dog, when the intermediate host is sheep, cattle, horse, or hog (Mediterranean, Middle East, New Zealand, and South America); or wolf, when the intermediate host is deer or moose (Canada and Alaska). In most cases, the disease is acquired in childhood. Organs affected include: liver (75%), lung (15%), peritoneum (10%), kidney (5%), and spleen (5%).

Most cysts are clinically silent but may present as abdominal pain, distension, or a mass. Recurrent jaundice and biliary colic may occur, due to the passage of cysts into the biliary tree, and cyst rupture may result in anaphylaxis and urticaria.

A blood eosinophilia is seen in 20 to 50% of cases. Other investigations include: immuno-electrophoresis (most specific), indirect haemaglutination test (85% sensitivity), complement fixation test (65% sensitivity), and Casoni test (60% sensitivity, with false positives found). The plain radiograph shows calcification (commonly crescent or ring shaped) in 10 to 30% of cases. CT is more sensitive for calcification and also shows the well-defined, low attenuation cyst (which may have internal septation). Enhancement of the cyst wall occurs after IV contrast. Ultrasound (Fig. 66a) most often shows a complex cyst of mixed echogenicity, with internal undulating membranes or a mass with peripheral calcification.

If percutaneous aspiration is performed, anaphylaxis occurs in 0.5% and asthma in 3%. The aspirated fluid gives a positive diagnosis in 70% of cases. Medical treatment may be with albendazole.

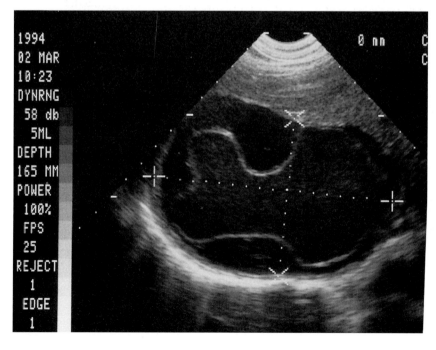

Fig. 66a Hydatid cyst. Hepatic ultrasound shows a cystic lesion with an internal membrane.

Question 67

This is an endoscopic retrograde cholangiopancreatogram (ERCP) performed on a 42-year-old man with epigastric and right upper quadrant pain and pruritis. Describe the abnormality. What is the most likely diagnosis? What associated intestinal condition may be present?

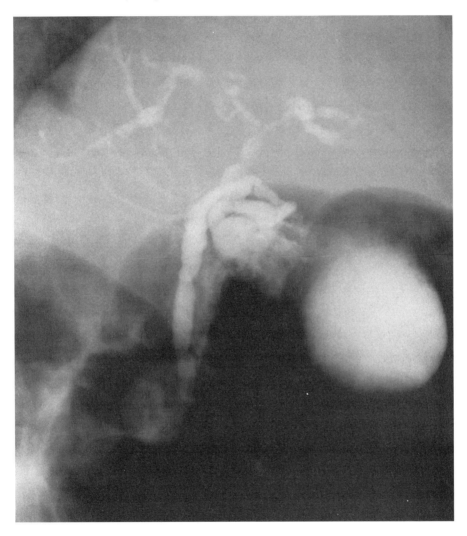

Fig. 67

Answer 67: Primary sclerosing cholangitis (PSC)

Findings: Multiple, irregular strictures of the intra- and extrahepatic biliary tree are present. This gives a 'beaded' and 'pruned-tree' appearance to the bile ducts.

Coincidental ulcerative colitis is found in 70% of patients with PSC. The PSC may precede the colitis. Areas of ductal normality exist between the ductal strictures and duct dilatation may be present upstream from strictures. The combination of strictures and dilatation gives the 'beaded' appearance which is typical of PSC. The strictures result from non-uniform chronic obliterative inflammatory fibrosis. Patients present with: chronic intermittent jaundice, fatigue, pruritus, right upper quadrant pain, and fever (30%). There is usually an elevated serum alkaline phosphatase, with mildly abnormal bilirubin and transaminase levels. PSC is a progressive process with a 5-year survival rate of 90% and a median survival time of 12 years.

Imaging is required to establish a firm diagnosis in many cases. ERCP is the most sensitive and specific study. Strictures vary in length from 1 mm to several cm. The common bile duct is almost always involved and the intra- and extrahepatic ducts are involved in combination in up to 90% of patients. Involvement of the gallbladder is seen in 15% and coincidental calculi are found in 25%. As the process progresses, peripheral ducts become obliterated and the appearance of the biliary tree is that of a 'pruned tree'. There may be 'diverticula' up to 10 mm in size (25%).

CT and ultrasound are less sensitive than ERCP but their advantage is that they demonstrate the entire biliary tree when a distal stricture prevents proximal biliary opacification at ERCP. CT identifies the complications of PSC (cirrhosis, portal hypertension, and cholangiocarcinoma); and shows bile duct wall thickening (when greater than 5 mm).

Question 68

This 58-year-old man presented with chronic epigastric pain and weight loss. What is the diagnosis?

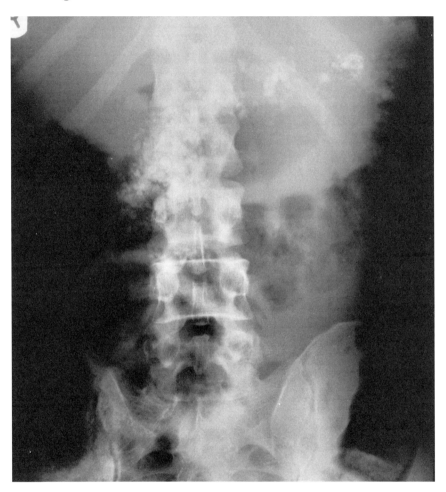

Fig. 68

Answer 68: Chronic pancreatitis

Findings: There is calcification across the upper abdomen in the position of the pancreas.

Chronic pancreatitis is less common than acute pancreatitis. There is prolonged inflammation leading to irreversible structural and functional changes within the pancreas. Risk factors for chronic pancreatitis include: alcohol consumption (75%), pancreas divisum, hyperparathyroidism, trauma, hyperlipidaemia, and, rarely, obstruction of the pancreatic duct. The characteristic symptoms are pain and weight loss. The major differential diagnosis is carcinoma of the pancreas. The pain is typically severe (requiring opiate analgesia) and epigastric, with radiation to the back. As the disease progresses, both the endocrine and exocrine components of the gland are destroyed resulting in diabetes mellitus and malabsorption. The typical calcification seen on the plain film is diagnostic of chronic pancreatitis, but is seen in only 40 to 60% of patients with alcohol induced disease (90% of patients with calcific pancreatitis have a history of alcoholism). Endoscopic retrograde cholangio-pancreatography (ERCP) demonstrates dilatation, irregularity, and stenosis of the branches of the main pancreatic duct branches in early disease. With disease progression, the main duct becomes involved. Intraductal calculi may also be seen.

Ultrasound is 75% accurate in the diagnosis of chronic pancreatitis. Abnormalities of the ducts, size/ morphology, and echogenicity are seen. Duct dilatation is the most specific finding (seen in up to 90%). The gland is usually atrophied (50%) in the chronic phase of the disease and has an irregular contour (60%). Pseudocysts may be present (25%). The CT features of chronic pancreatitis are similar to those found on ultrasound but CT may also demonstrate complications such as portal/ splenic vein thrombosis. The unenhanced CT (Fig. 68a) demonstrates pancreatic calcification (arrowheads) with an intraductal calculus (curved arrow) in the pancreatic head.

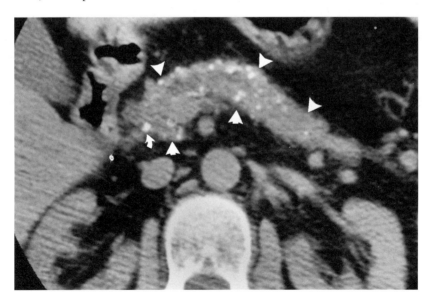

Fig. 68a   Unenhanced CT showing chronic pancreatitis.

Question 69

This is an axial contrast enhanced CT section through the liver and spleen of a 46-year-old woman with a history of chronic alcoholism. What is the underlying hepatic process and what complication has occurred?

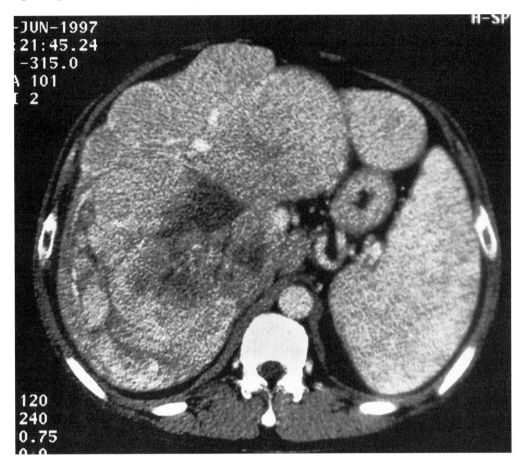

Fig. 69

Answer 69: Hepatic cirrhosis complicated by the development of hepatocellular carcinoma (HCC)

Findings: The liver edge is irregular with nodular regeneration consistent with cirrhosis (arrowheads, Fig. 69a). Superimposed on this cirrhotic change is a low density area (arrows) with ill-defined margins which is a hepatoma. Invasion of the portal vein has occurred (between curved arrows). Splenomegaly (S) secondary to portal hypertension is also present.

World-wide, HCC is the most frequent primary visceral tumour. It accounts for 90% of primary liver malignancies and has an incidence ranging from <1% in the industrialized world to 20% in areas of south-east Asia and Africa. In developed countries, the peak age range is 50 to 60. In the high incidence areas, the peak age is 30 to 40. The tumour may be diffuse microscopic (50%), solitary (30%), or multifocal nodular (20%). HCC most commonly occurs secondary to alcohol or hepatitis B induced cirrhosis. It may also be related to carcinogens (aflatoxin, anabolic steroids, and oral contraceptives) and metabolic errors (haemochromatosis, tyrosinosis, galactosaemia, and type I glycogen storage disease). Presentation is variable and includes: fever, malaise, weight loss, right upper quadrant pain, hepatomegaly, ascites, and a paraneoplastic syndrome. The α-fetoprotein is elevated in 90% of cases. Imaging is central to the confirmation of HCC, and ultrasound and CT are initially performed. A high degree of suspicion is required if small lesions are not to be missed. The features vary with the tumour type. Intra-arterial CT portography, CT after iodized oil injection (lipiodol), and intraoperative ultrasound are the most sensitive ways of identifying HCC, particularly if the lesion is less than 3 cm in diameter. Imaging guided chemotherapeutic embolization or injection of alcohol into the tumour may be of use in management, reducing tumour size prior to surgery.

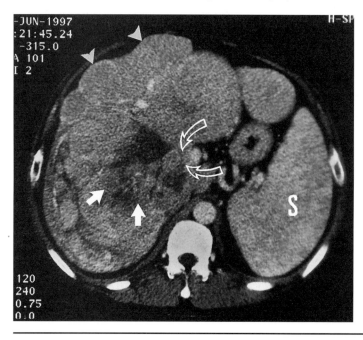

Fig. 69a   CT showing hepatocellular carcinoma complicating cirrhosis.

Question 70

This 57-year-old woman presented with acute on chronic epigastric pain, jaundice, and fever. The ultrasound image shows a longitudinal section of the extrahepatic common bile duct (cephalad is to the left of the image). What is the diagnosis?

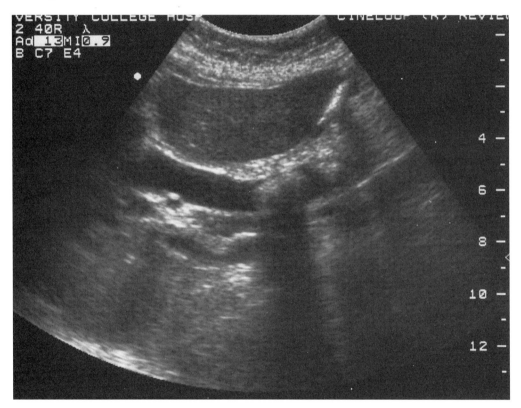

Fig. 70

Answer 70: Obstructive jaundice due to a biliary calculus in the common bile duct

Findings: Using the liver (L) as an acoustic window (Fig. 70a), the common bile duct (arrows) is seen to be occluded at its lower end by an echogenic mass (calculus, arrowheads) which is casting an acoustic shadow.

The incidence of gallbladder calculi is 10% and increases with age. M:F ratio is 1:3. The calculi may be pure cholesterol (10%), predominantly cholesterol (with calcium carbonate/bilirubinate, 70%), or pigment (20%). Predisposing and associated conditions include: haemolytic disease, for example sickle cell and spherocytosis; inflammatory bowel disease; and metabolic disorders, for example diabetes mellitus. In patients with gallbladder calculi, 66% are asymptomatic. Once biliary symptoms have occurred, there is a 50% chance of recurrence within 1 year and a 1 to 2% chance of developing acute cholecystitis per year.

Ultrasound is the investigation of choice with sensitivity and specificity for diagnosing gallstones in excess of 95%. It is important that the gallbladder is studied in the fasting state.

Common bile duct calculi most commonly originated in the gallbladder; 15% of patients undergoing cholecystectomy for calculus disease have bile duct calculi. However, 10% of patients with bile duct calculi are found not to have gallbladder calculi. Calculi less than 6 mm in diameter usually pass spontaneously. Ultrasound is the investigation of choice in patients suspected of having biliary tree calculi but calculi are only seen in about 50%. ERCP may then be needed; at the time of the procedure a therapeutic sphincterotomy may be performed for gallstone extraction.

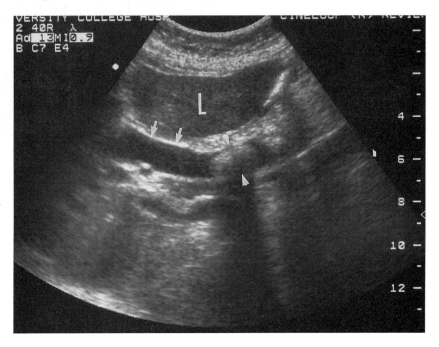

Fig. 70a   Common bile duct obstruction due to a calculus.

Question 71

This patient presented with severe epigastric pain. What is the diagnosis and what complications are present? What predisposing factors are there to this condition?

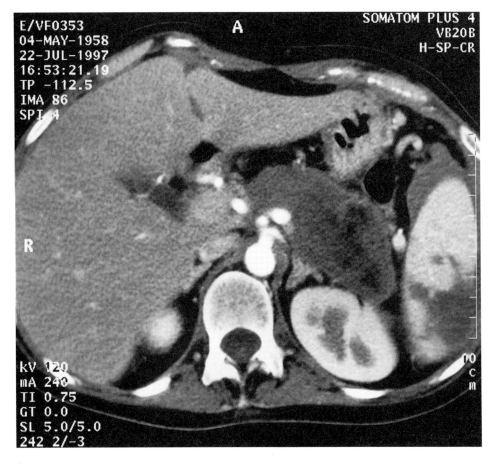

Fig. 71

Answer 71: Acute pancreatitis

Findings: The pancreas (P) is diffusely oedematous with focal areas of inflammation or necrosis consistent with severe acute pancreatitis. Splenic infarction (straight black arrow, Fig. 71a), portal vein thrombosis (curved arrow), and ascites (straight white arrow) are complications seen on this image.

Acute pancreatitis has many aetiologies. Alcoholism and biliary calculi account for up to 90% of cases. Other causes include: metabolic disorders, for example hypercalcaemia and hyperlipidaemia; infection, for example mumps; trauma; drugs, for example steroids; and congenital abnormalities. The serum amylase and lipase only show elevated levels in 80 to 90% of cases and the degree of elevation does not correlate well with the severity of the inflammatory process. Fifty percent of cases are mild while 10% of cases are severe leading to death from sepsis, respiratory, or renal failure.

A wide range of imaging investigations may be abnormal. A chest film shows pleural effusion, basal atelectasis, diaphragmatic elevation, pulmonary air space opacity, or adult respiratory distress syndrome (ARDS). An abdominal film most commonly shows an abnormality of the intestinal gas pattern. This may be duodenal ileus (40%), a sentinel loop, or paucity of gas in the colon distal to the splenic flexure. Inflammatory masses may be identified. Ultrasound can demonstrate acute pancreatitis, but is less sensitive/ specific than CT. Its main use is as a screening tool for biliary calculi or following a known abnormality in patients with more severe disease. CT is the investigation of choice in patients with more severe disease, where there is a diagnostic dilemma or where complications such as pseudo-cyst infection, haemorrhage, pancreatic necrosis, or aneurysm formation are suspected.

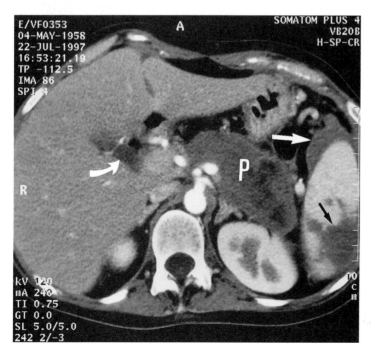

Fig. 71a   Enhanced CT showing acute pancreatitis.

Question 72

This is the contrast enhanced axial CT of a 66-year-old man with a 3-month history of weight loss. What abnormality is present? What is the most likely source?

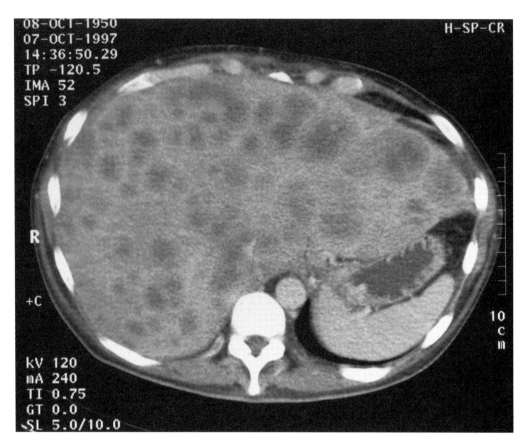

Fig. 72

Answer 72: Liver metastases

Findings: Multiple areas of low attenuation are seen in the liver.

Multiple focal liver lesions may be benign (simple cysts, polycystic disease, abscesses, haemangiomata, adenomata, regenerating nodules, and Caroli's disease) or malignant (metastases, multifocal hepatocellular carcinoma, and lymphoma). Metastases are the most common malignant liver lesion. They are multiple in 98% of cases. The most common primary sites are: colon, stomach, pancreas, breast, and lung.

The clinical features of metastatic disease are rarely specific. Only 50% of patients dying with hepatic deposits have symptoms or signs directly referable to the liver. These include: hepatomegaly (30%), ascites (20%), and jaundice (15%). Analysis of liver function is also non-specific. Up to 50% of patients with metastases have normal liver function tests and in patients with an abnormality the profile will frequently not differentiate metastases from obstruction to the biliary tree by tumour mass or chemotherapeutic hepatotoxicity. Imaging is essential for the diagnosis of liver metastases but biopsy is still required for histological confirmation of the nature of a hepatic lesion.

The imaging features of liver metastases on ultrasound, CT, and MRI are highly variable.

Question 73

This 55-year-old man was admitted with a blood pressure of 75/50 mmHg. What is the diagnosis and give three causes?

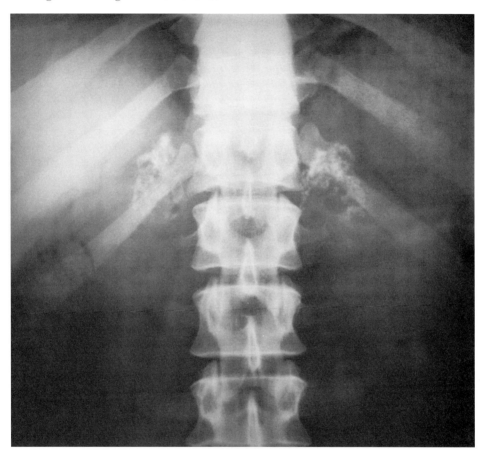

Fig. 73

Answer 73: Addisonian crisis

Findings: There is bilateral adrenal calcification.

Causes of adrenal calcification are:

(1)   autoimmune (Addison's disease)—the commonest cause;

(2)   infective—tuberculosis, histoplasmosis;

(3)   neoplasms—adenoma, carcinoma (irregular punctate calcification), neuroblastoma (50% ill-defined calcification), phaeochromocytoma (eggshell calcification), and metastases;

(4)   haemorrhage secondary to birth trauma, infection, or arterial/ venous thrombosis;

(5)   Wolman's disease—a rare autosomal recessive lipoidosis with hepatosplenomegaly and adrenomegaly.

An addisonian crisis is a medical emergency and requires immediate repletion of the intravascular space with intravenous saline, colloids, and steroids. A precipitating factor should be sought such as infection or myocardial infarction. The diagnosis may be confirmed by a short synacthen test.

Question 74

This 64-year-old female presented with generalized abdominal distension. What abnormality is shown on this ultrasound image? List four causes.

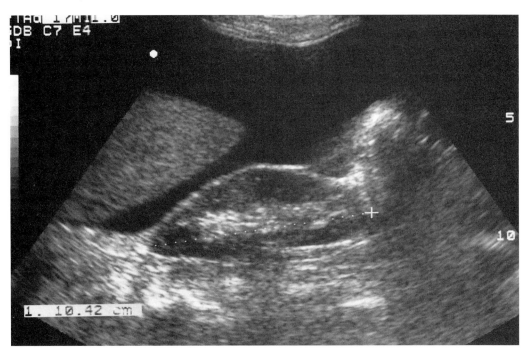

Fig. 74

Answer 74: Ascites

Findings: The liver and right kidney are separated by anechoic ascitic fluid (black). The right kidney has been measured.

Clear fluid presents no acoustic interfaces to the ultrasound beam and is therefore echo-free (anechoic). Ascitic fluid may be a transudate (due to congestive cardiac failure, constrictive pericarditis, hypoproteinaemia, chronic renal failure, cirrhosis, or Budd–Chiari syndrome), an exudate (malignant, part of a poly-serositis, infective, or inflammatory), haemorrhagic, or chylous.

Patients with ascites may initially be asymptomatic; develop a sensation of fullness and distension, or anorexia, nausea, vomiting, pain, or respiratory distress with a large amount of ascites.

Physical examination may reveal as little as 300 ml of ascitic fluid, but can be difficult even with 2 litres of fluid present. Flank bulging and shifting dullness (most sensitive sign) and a fluid thrill (most specific sign) may be found.

Ultrasound accurately identifies any ascites. A diagnostic paracentesis may be performed to aid diagnosis. Transudates (protein of <25 g/l and a specific gravity of <1016) can be distinguished from exudates. A polymorphonuclear white cell count of >250/mm^3 suggests pyogenic infection or acute pancreatitis. A pH of <7.35 is found with neoplasia, infection, and pancreatitis. An amylase of >1000 IU/l (and a protein >30 g/l) indicates pancreatitis.

NEPHROLOGY

Question 75

What does this intravenous urogram show?

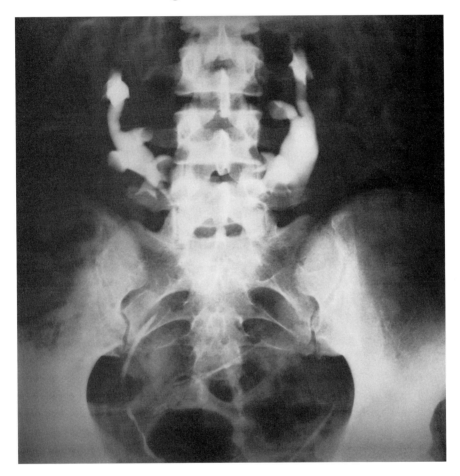

Fig. 75

Answer 75: Horseshoe kidney

Findings: The lower poles of the kidneys are united by a bridge of tissue, which is parenchymal in 90% and fibrous tissue in 10%. The kidneys are lower in the abdomen than usual. The orientation of the kidneys is abnormal, the lower poles being more medially sited than the upper poles.

Horseshoe kidneys have an incidence of 0.2 to 1% and a male predominance (male: female 2:1). Horseshoe kidney is associated with cardiovascular and skeletal anomalies, anorectal malformation, genitourinary anomalies (hypospadia, undescended testis, bicornuate uterus, and ureteral duplication), trisomy 18, and Turner's syndrome.

The pelvi–ureteric junction faces anteriorly instead of medially and so the ureter has to run anteriorly to cross the joining bridge between the kidneys. This impairs urinary drainage so there is an increased incidence of obstruction and calculi. Horseshoe kidneys also have an increased incidence of vesicoureteric reflux and Wilms tumour. There is an increased susceptibility to trauma as horseshoe kidneys are more superficial and overlie the lumbar spine.

Question 76

This 60-year-old lady presented with left loin pain, fevers, and rigors. What is the diagnosis and what underlying disorder is commonly associated?

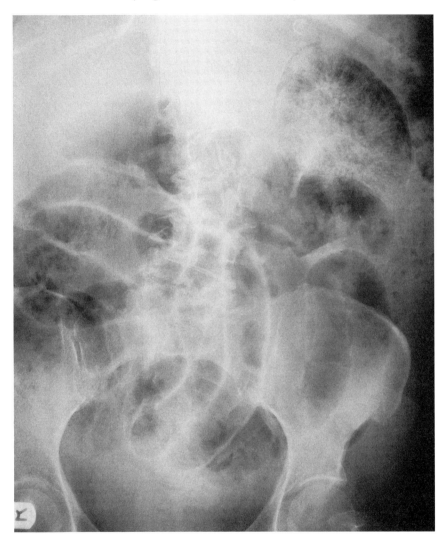

Fig. 76

Answer 76: Emphysematous pyelonephritis, diabetes mellitus is found in approximately 90%

Findings: A gas-filled lesion is seen in the region of the left kidney with streaks of gas in the renal parenchyma radiating from the medulla to cortex. Gas is also seen within the collecting system. There is an associated ileus with dilated gas filled loops of small bowel.

Emphysematous pyelonephritis is a fulminant infection of the kidney. Abscess formation is associated with gas in a non-functioning kidney and in the perirenal tissues.

The causative organism is usually *E. coli* or *Proteus* and rarely *Clostridia*. The condition occurs in diabetic and immunocompromised patients. Renal obstruction occurs in 40% of patients. It is commoner in females. An axial CT (Fig. 76a) shows complete disruption of the left kidney (curved arrows) associated with a gaseous abscess (arrowheads) and some free peritoneal fluid (straight arrow). The mortality is high (40 to 50%). The management is intravenous antibiotics and prompt drainage via a nephrostomy, performed under fluoroscopic or ultrasound guidance.

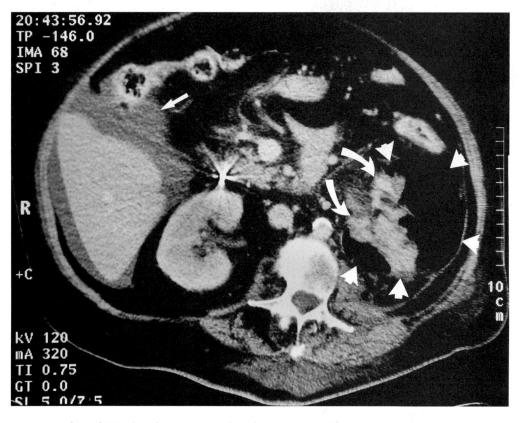

Fig. 76a   Enhanced CT of emphysematous pyelonephritis.

Question 77

This 36-year-old alcoholic gave a history of recurrent loin pain. A control film showed no renal tract calcification. What does the intravenous urogram show?

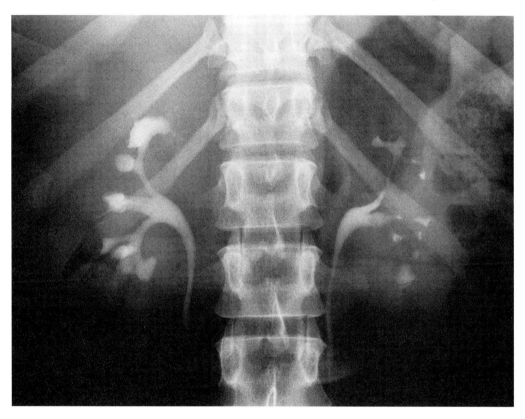

Fig. 77

Answer 77: Papillary necrosis

Findings: The calyces are blunted and mildly dilated. The features are best demonstrated in the right kidney. Some contrast medium is seen outside the calyces, in the papillae (upper pole of right kidney). The right renal cortical outline is smooth.

There are various phases of papillary necrosis on an intravenous urogram. The earliest phase is enlargement of the papilla (papillary swelling), followed by fine projections of contrast medium along the papilla or entering the papillary tip. The papilla then shrinks with partial, then complete, detachment. In partial detachment, the pyramid and papilla resemble an 'egg in cup' appearance. The papilla may then slough off and may: (1) be passed in the urine, (2) cause ureteric obstruction, (3) remain free in the calyx, or (4) remain in the renal pelvis and calcify. The calyces appear dilated following papillary sloughing.

The pathogenesis is ischaemia of the medulla secondary to interstitial nephritis (interstitial oedema) or intrinsic vascular obstruction. The following are recognized causes: diabetes mellitus, sickle cell disease, analgesic abuse, pyelonephritis, obstruction with infection, alcohol abuse, infantile dehydration, and renal vein thrombosis. There is an increased incidence of squamous cell carcinoma and transitional cell carcinoma of the renal pelvis in analgesic abusers.

Question 78

This 26-year-old girl presented with chronic renal impairment. A control film showed no renal tract calcification. The intravenous urogram 20 min post injection is shown. What is the most likely cause of the renal impairment?

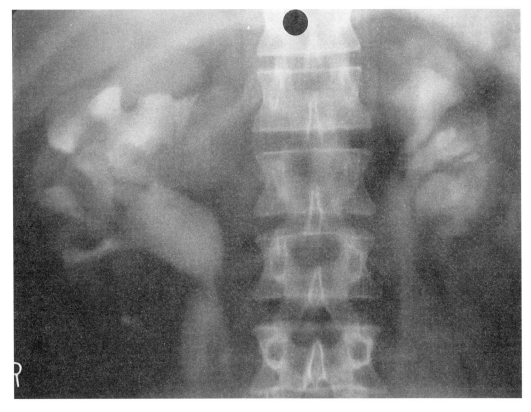

Fig. 78

Answer 78: Reflux nephropathy

Findings: The intravenous urogram shows bilateral small kidneys with clubbed calyces. Scarring of the cortex opposite the clubbed calyces is seen.

Vesicoureteric reflux is most commonly idiopathic in children. It may resolve as the child ages. When reflux is combined with infection and intrarenal reflux, nephron loss and scar formation opposite the clubbed calyx ensues. Intrarenal reflux of infected urine predominately occurs at the poles of the kidneys because compound papillas favour reflux when compared to the simple papillae of the interpolar calyces.

Reflux can be diagnosed by either a micturating cystogram or by a radionuclide micturating cystogram which has a lower ionizing radiation dose. Screening of siblings is recommended because of the increased incidence of reflux in them.

Question 79

What is the most likely diagnosis and what urogenital complications may occur?

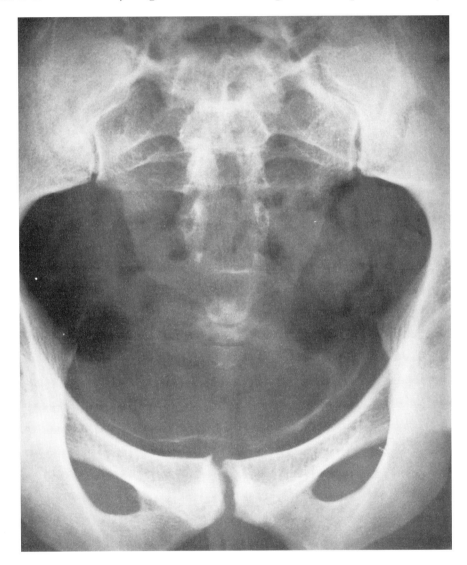

Fig. 79

Answer 79: Schistosomiasis

Complications: Ureteric strictures in the distal third of the ureter, urethral strictures with perineal fistulae, vesicoureteric reflux, squamous carcinoma of the bladder, and ureteric dilatation secondary to fibrosis.

Findings: There is curvilinear calcification of the bladder wall. The appearances are virtually pathognomonic of schistosomiasis.

Other causes of bladder wall calcification include: tuberculosis, transitional and squamous cell carcinoma, and cyclophosphamide-induced cystitis. Tuberculosis usually results in a small contracted bladder with calcification elsewhere in the urogenital tract. Unlike schistosomiasis, the disease starts in the kidney and spreads distally.

S. haematobium is the commonest *Schistosomiasis* sp. to affect the urogenital tract. The disease is endemic in parts of Africa. The water snail is the intermediate host, with the cercaria stage penetrating the human skin (usually the foot) and travelling via the lymphatics to the portal and pelvic venous plexuses. The adults live in the pelvic venous plexus where the female sheds eggs which erode the walls of the bladder and ureter and are passed into the urine or produce fibrosis and calcification within the wall. The diagnosis is made by detecting the eggs in the stools, urine, or in a rectal biopsy. Praziquantel is the drug therapy of choice.

Question 80

This is a bilateral retrograde pyelogram performed on a 40-year-old lady with a history of renal stones. What is the diagnosis?

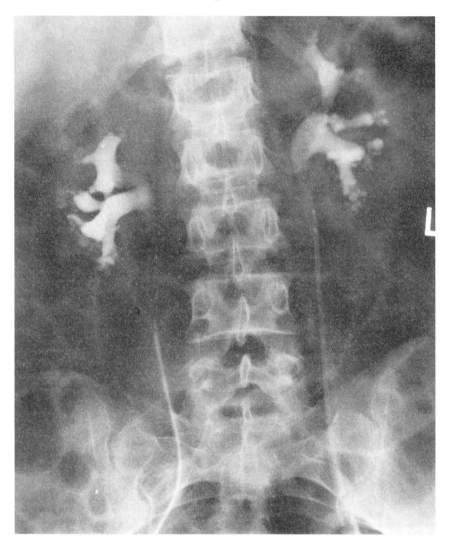

Fig. 80

Answer 80: Medullary sponge kidney

Findings: Bilateral ureteric catheters are present. Multiple rounded and linear opacities extend from the renal papillas into the medulla. These represent contrast filling, dilated ectatic collecting tubules (bunch of grapes appearance). The precontrast film showed some of these tubules to contain small calculi.

Medullary sponge kidney is a sporadic condition which may be asymptomatic and is often a chance finding on an intravenous urogram. It is characterized by dysplastic cystic dilatation of papillary and medullary portions of the collecting ducts. The aetiology is unknown. Calculi form within the ectatic collecting tubules due to urinary stasis and give a bunch of grapes appearance. A calculus may pass down the ureter causing colic and obstruction. Patients also present with recurrent pyelonephritis or haematuria. The condition is associated with hepatic fibrosis, skeletal hemihypertrophy, parathyroid adenoma, Caroli disease, and Ehlers–Danlos syndrome. The condition is unilateral in 25% and may involve only one pyramid.

Question 81

This 55-year-old patient presented with chronic back pain and weight loss. The intravenous urogram (IVU) 90 min postinjection is shown. The control film showed no renal tract calcification. What is the diagnosis?

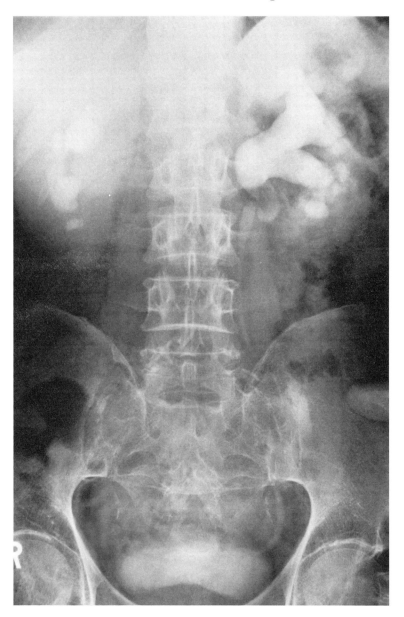

Fig. 81

Answer 81: Retroperitoneal fibrosis (RPF)

Findings: The IVU shows bilateral, dilated pelvicalyceal systems with dilatation of the proximal left ureter. The obstruction is partial as contrast is seen in the left distal ureter and bladder.

The differential of bilateral renal obstruction is wide but includes prostatic disease, gynaecological malignancies, and bilateral renal tract calculi. The IVU can define the level of obstruction and the cause may be ascertained by ultrasound or CT with biopsy (Fig. 81a).

In RPF, fibrous tissue exerts its effects on the ureters, great vessels, and lymphatics. The primary form (66%) is probably autoimmune in aetiology and is associated with mediastinal fibrosis, sclerosing cholangitis, Riedel's thyroiditis, and retro-orbital pseudotumour. It is responsive to steroids.

Secondary RPF (33%) may be due to:

(1) drugs—methysergide;
(2) tumours—lymphoma, retroperitoneal metastases (breast, colon), carcinoid;
(3) inflammatory conditions—trauma, surgery, infection, Crohn's disease, and pancreatitis;
(4) aortic aneurysm (desmoplastic response);
(5) connective tissue disease—polyarteritis nodosa.

Clinical features of both forms include renal obstruction (50 to 60%), back pain (90%), an elevated erythrocyte sedimentation rate (ESR), peripheral oedema, and fever. CT is useful in delineating the extent of retroperitoneal fibrosis and the structures involved. Fig. 81a depicts the retroperitoneal mass (arrows) surrounding the aorta (arrowhead). A left ureteric stent (black arrow) is present. The fibrosis rarely extends below the pelvic brim but may extend cranially into the mediastinum. Management is withdrawal of any causative factor, relief of the renal obstruction, and steroids.

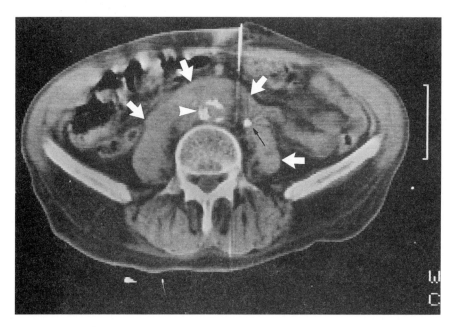

Fig. 81a Axial CT through the lower abdomen of a different patient undergoing CT guided biopsy of a retroperitoneal mass (lymphoma).

Question 82

This is an intravenous urogram (IVU) performed on a 50-year-old patient with hypertension. The control film showed no renal tract calcification. What is the diagnosis?

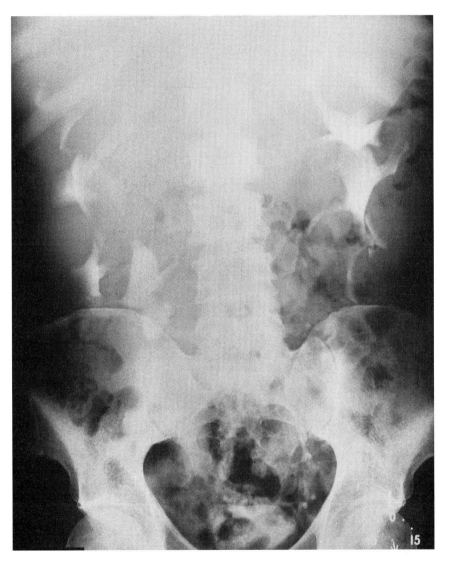

Fig. 82

Answer 82: Adult polycystic kidney disease

Findings: The kidneys are enlarged with spidery distorted pelvicalyceal systems due to multiple cysts.

The condition is inherited in an autosomal dominant manner. The renal cysts, which may be present at birth, progressively increase in size with compression and loss of the normal intervening renal tissue such that patients may present from the fourth decade onwards with chronic renal failure, haematuria, or abdominal pain. Hepatic cysts are seen in 30% of patients without liver dysfunction (Fig. 82a(i). Cysts may also occur in the pancreas, spleen, and other organs. Berry aneurysms of the cerebral vessels are also associated. The renal cysts may be complicated by haemorrhage (with loin pain and haematuria), calculus formation, infection, cyst rupture, or development of renal cell carcinoma. Ultrasound and CT are useful in the imaging of the complications. Formerly, the condition was diagnosed by IVU but is now screened for by ultrasound (Fig. 82a(ii). This is performed at age 20 years as the condition may be difficult to exclude before this age.

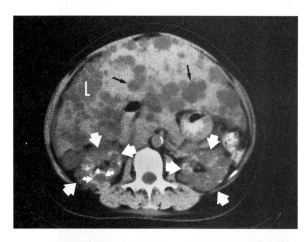

Fig. 82a(i)   Contrast enhanced CT through the liver (L) and polycystic kidneys (white arrows). There are multiple hepatic (black arrows) and renal cysts (curved arrows).

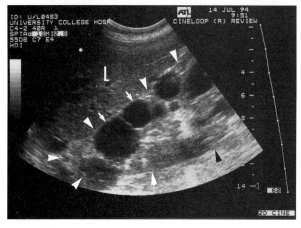

Fig. 82a(ii)   Ultrasound using the liver (L) as a window to image the right kidney (outline of right kidney indicated by arrowheads) which shows multiple cysts (arrows).

Question 83

This 55-year-old man presented with painless haematuria. A coronal T1 weighted MRI of the abdomen is shown; the liver (L) is indicated. What is the diagnosis and what complication has occurred?

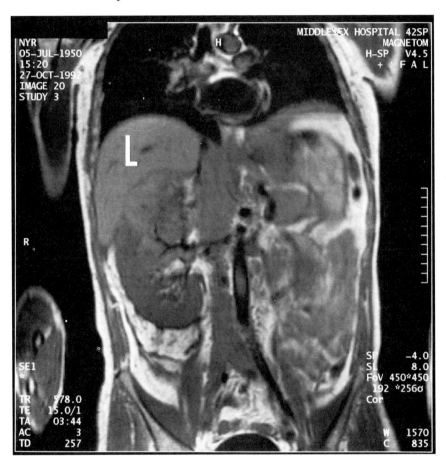

Fig. 83

Answer 83: Right renal cell carcinoma with thrombosis of the inferior vena cava

Findings: There is a mass in the upper pole of the right kidney of mixed signal (arrowheads, Fig. 83a), which histologically was a renal cell carcinoma. Extension of the tumour into the inferior vena cava (IVC) is demonstrated (arrows) resulting in thrombosis. Normally flowing blood is seen as a signal void on MR, that is black, as in the aorta to the left of the IVC.

Renal cell carcinoma (hypernephroma) make up 80 to 90% of all primary renal malignancies. The peak age of presentation is 55 years and it is more common in males. Predisposing conditions include: von Hippel–Lindau disease, acquired cystic disease of uraemia, and angiomyolipomas (associated with tuberous sclerosis). Five to 10% are bilateral. Renal cell carcinoma presents with haematuria (56%), loin pain due to clot colic (36%), pyrexia of unknown origin (<5%), varicocele (2%), or as an incidental renal mass. Presentation may also be with paraneoplastic syndromes with polycythaemia and hypercalcaemia since erythropoietin, parathormone, and vitamin D metabolites may be secreted. Metastases are most commonly to lung, seen as cannon ball metastases (55%), lymph nodes (34%), and bones (expanded and lytic) in 32%. On an intravenous urogram hypernephromas show displacement and distortion of calyces and renal pelvis. Non-excretion of contrast is seen in renal vein invasion. Ultrasound (US) is the initial investigation of choice with the majority of tumours appearing hyperechoic. Renal vein and IVC patency can be assessed on ultrasound. CT is then indicated for staging purposes. Angiography no longer plays the central role it once did, having been superseded by US and CT. MRI is useful in assessing IVC patency and for staging where iodinated contrast is contraindicated. The treatment is nephrectomy. The 5-year survival exceeds 50%.

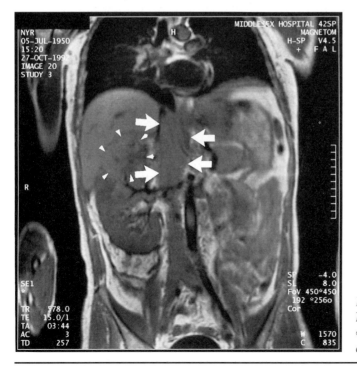

Fig. 83a   Coronal T1 weighted MRI showing a renal cell carcinoma with extension into the inferior vena cava (IVC).

Question 84

This 28-year-old lady was found to be hypertensive. This is an aortogram with the right renal artery labelled. What is the diagnosis?

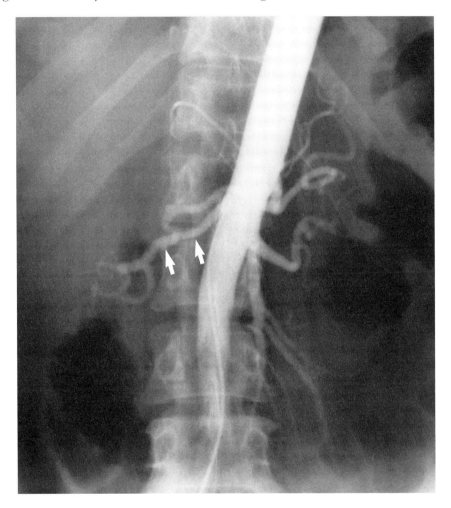

Fig. 84

Answer 84: *Fibromuscular dysplasia of the right renal artery*

Findings: There are alternating segments of stenosis and ectasia along the right renal artery. The appearance has been described as a 'string of beads'.

Fibromuscular dysplasia (FMD) accounts for 35% of renal artery stenoses, with atherosclerosis being the major cause in the older age group (65%). It is the commonest cause of renovascular hypertension in young adults. It is commoner in females (M:F 1:3), bilateral in 60% with a higher right sided incidence (R:L 4:1). The mid and distal main renal artery is involved in 79% of cases with sparing of the proximal third in 98%. In contrast, atheromatous renal artery stenosis usually affects the proximal 2 cm. Other aortic branches may be involved in 1 to 2%. Children may be affected by the disease. FMD is subdivided into medial fibroplasia (60 to 70%), as shown in this case, perimedial fibroplasia (15 to 25%—seen as long irregular stenoses with beading), medial hyperplasia (5 to 15%—long smooth narrowing), medial dissection (5%—aneurysms and false channels), intimal fibroplasia (1 to 2%—focal stenosis), and adventitial fibroplasia (<1%—long segmental stenosis). Complications include giant aneurysms and arteriovenous fistulae between the renal artery and vein in medial fibroplasia. Management is by transluminal balloon angioplasty which has a 90% success rate with a low rate of restenosis. Resection of the affected segment can also be performed with end-to-end anastomosis.

Question 85

This 35-year-old man presented with a 48-hour history of left loin pain. What does this renal ultrasound show and what is the diagnosis?

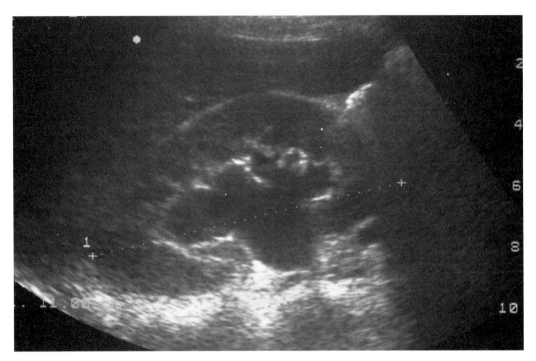

Fig. 85

Answer 85: Obstruction of the left kidney

Findings: There is dilatation of the left pelvicalyceal (PC) system due to obstruction by a stone (not shown).

Dilatation of the urinary tract is the hallmark of obstructive uropathy but whilst it is strongly suggestive of obstruction, it is not diagnostic. The absence of PC dilatation in early obstruction and dehydrated states and its presence without obstruction are obvious exceptions.

Imaging modalities vary in the amount of anatomical and functional information they provide. Ultrasonography (US) provides anatomical detail but little functional information. US is the modality of choice in the initial investigation and often demonstrates the cause and level of obstruction. The proximal and distal ureter is usually well visualized but the middle third of the ureter is difficult to image. If the policy that PC dilatation equates with obstruction is adopted, a false positive rate of up to 20% can be expected. Intravenous urography (IVU) provides functional information as well as anatomical detail about the degree, level, and cause of obstruction. Computed tomography (CT) is challenging US as the initial investigation because of its ability to demonstrate retroperitoneal structures. Radionuclide studies offer more functional information than either IVU, US, or CT, but give poorer anatomical detail. Percutaneous nephrostomy is indicated in obstruction in the presence of a pyonephrosis, severe loin pain, and in order to preserve renal function.

Question 86

This 23-year-old lady presented with right loin pain. The 15-minute intravenous urogram (IVU) is shown. The control film was normal. What would you do next? What is the diagnosis?

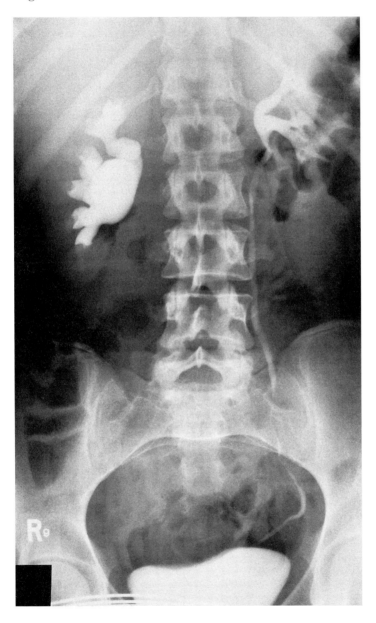

Fig. 86

Answer 86: Right pelviureteric junction (PUJ) obstruction

An intravenous frusemide (20 mg) challenge should be performed to differentiate from a baggy renal pelvis. In PUJ obstruction, this would induce a diuresis causing further dilatation of the right pelvicalyceal system confirming the diagnosis.

Findings: The right pelvicalyceal system is markedly dilated and no contrast is seen in the ureter. The left kidney is normal.

The aetiology of PUJ obstruction is unknown, but there is an associated aberrant lower pole vessel in 25% of patients. It can present at any age, is more common in males, and on the left side. Bilateral disease is seen in 25%. PUJ obstruction may be intermittent making diagnosis and response to therapy difficult to ascertain. Patients present with loin pain exacerbated by a diuresis. The IVU shows a dilated pelvicalyceal system with no ureteric filling and frusemide induces further dilatation and loin pain. The degree of obstruction is assessed by diuresis renography or upper tract urodynamics. Complications include loss of renal function, pyonephrosis, and haematuria. Treatment is by pyeloplasty or balloon dilatation.

MUSCULOSKELETAL

Question 87

This 20-year-old man presented with a painful left shoulder. What is the most likely diagnosis?

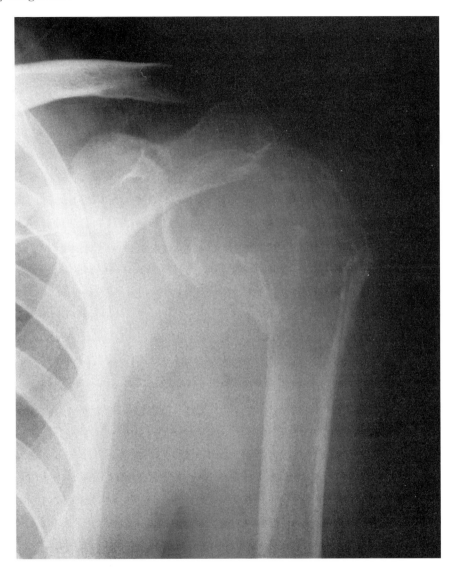

Fig. 87

Answer 87: Osteosarcoma

Findings: There is an aggressive lytic process affecting the left humeral head with cortical destruction and a Codman's triangle type periosteal reaction. The glenoid is not involved. The distal extent of the bony involvement is ill-defined ('wide zone of transition') indicative of an aggressive process. There is an associated soft tissue mass. The differential would include; an osteomyelitis (typically metaphyseal and may have an associated septic arthritis) or a Ewing's sarcoma (typically diaphyseal with an 'onion-skin' periosteal reaction).

Osteosarcoma is the most common primary malignant bone tumour in childhood, occurring between 15 and 25 years in 75% of cases. There is a predilection for long bones, especially around the knee. Imaging plays an important role in staging. MRI (Fig. 87a) is the modality of choice for assessing local spread as it is very sensitive in delineating marrow involvement (black arrowheads), extension into adjacent soft tissues (curved white arrows), and in assessing response to therapy. As part of the staging work-up, patients also have a radionuclide bone scan (to look for skeletal metastases) and a chest radiograph and a CT chest to identify pulmonary metastases. However, biopsy of the primary lesion is essential to obtain histological grade.

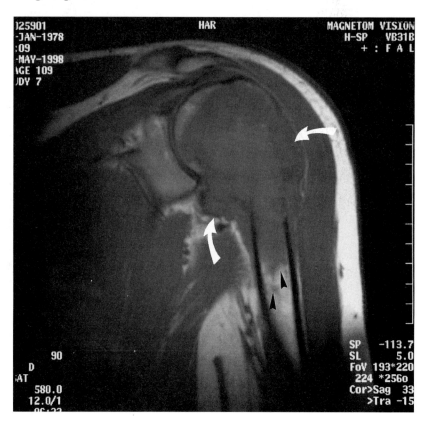

Fig. 87a   Coronal T1 weighted MRI showing an osteosarcoma of the proximal humerus.

Question 88

This 42-year-old man gave an acute history of right loin pain superimposed on a long history of back pain.

1. State three abnormalities on this intravenous urogram (IVU).
2. What is the underlying diagnosis?

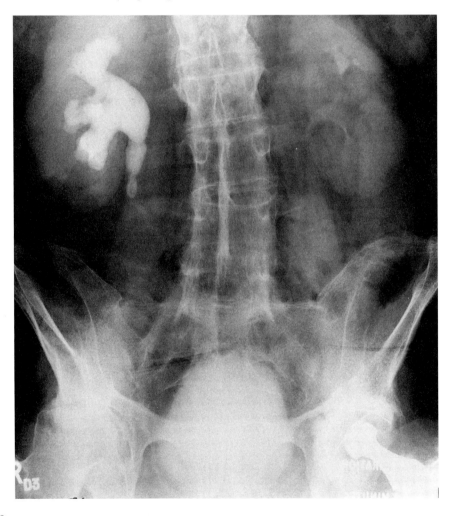

Fig. 88

Answer 88: Ankylosing spondylitis

(1) Abnormalities are:
   (a) bilateral bony ankylosis of the sacroiliac joints;
   (b) ankylosis of the posterior neural arches, interspinous ligaments, and several discs (bamboo spine),
   (c) obstruction of the right kidney due to a renal calculus in the proximal ureter—renal calculi are not known to be associated with ankylosing spondylitis but possible aetiologies in this case are hypercalcuria, urinary stasis, or a sloughed calcified papilla due to papillary necrosis induced by analgesic abuse;
   (d) there is loss of the hip joint space on the right and irregularity of the femoral head consistent with an arthropathy—a left hip prosthesis is present.

(2) The diagnosis is ankylosing spondylitis.

The diagnosis is made from the following radiological features:

1. Bilateral sacroiliitis (essential) characterized initially by bony erosions followed by ankylosis.

2. Spinal involvement—squaring of the lumbar vertebrae (osteitis), annulus fibrosus ossification resulting in syndesmophyte formation, ossification of the interspinous ligaments and ankylosis of the apophyseal, costotransverse and costovertebral joints. The classic 'bamboo spine' appearance is the end result. Similar changes are seen in the cervical spine.

3. Erosions followed by soft tissue ossification are seen at the sites of attachment of ligaments, tendons, and joint capsules to bone. The process is known as enthesopathy and sites commonly affected are the iliac crests, ischial tuberosities, and greater trochanters.

4. Hip and shoulder involvement, which is mild and transient in up to 50%. It may be aggressive with subchondral bone sclerosis, and cartilage ossification leading to bony ankylosis.

5. Apical lung fibrosis with cavitation.

Question 89

This Greek patient presented with chronic dyspnoea. What is the diagnosis and what other radiological features may be found elsewhere?

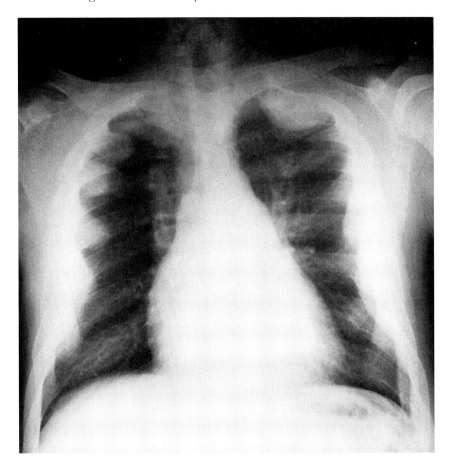

Fig. 89

Answer 89: Thalassemia major

Findings: The ribs are expanded with thinned cortices due to marrow hyperplasia. The heart size is enlarged consistent with a cardiomyopathy secondary to iron overload.

Other radiological features of thalassemia major are:

1. Skull—widening of the diploic space with coarsened trabeculas with a hair-on-end appearance. Also there is under pneumatization of the maxillary antra. These features are due to marrow hyperplasia.
2. Appendicular skeleton—widened medullary spaces with cortical thinning and osteoporosis. The normally concave ends of the long bones are convex (Erlenmeyer flask deformity). Premature epiphyseal fusion. An arthropathy due to pyrophosphate or urate deposition may be present. There is an increase in fractures.
3. Extramedullary haemopoiesis—paravertebral masses of haemopoietic tissue may be seen.
4. Abdomen—hepatosplenomegaly and gallstones. Iron overload in the liver is seen as low signal on T1 weighted MR images.

Question 90

This 55-year-old lady complained of long-standing abdominal pain and constipation. This is a magnified view of the right thumb and fingers. Name three abnormalities and what is the underlying diagnosis?

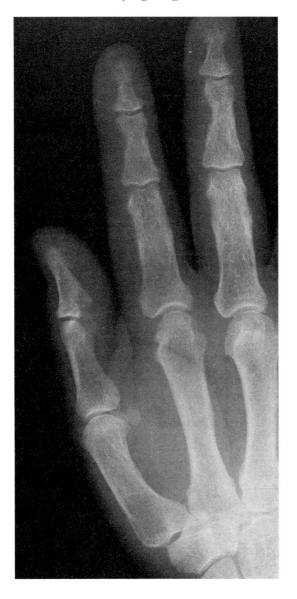

Fig. 90

Answer 90: Primary hyperparathyroidism

Abnormalities are:

(1)   terminal phalangeal tuft resorption;
(2)   subperiosteal bone erosion;
(3)   a lytic lesion at the base of the right first metacarpal ('brown tumour').

Subperiosteal bone resorption is pathognomonic of hyperparathyroidism and typically occurs on the radial aspect of the proximal and middle phalanges of the hand. Bony resorption is also seen at the distal phalangeal tufts, lateral ends of the clavicles, and lamina dura around the teeth. A 'brown tumour' (osteoclastoma) is due to parathormone (PTH) induced osteoclastic activity and occurs more commonly in primary than secondary hyperparathyroidism. The skull radiograph is described as pepper pot in appearance due to the irregular demineralization. Presenting complaints include bone pain, abdominal pain due to constipation, renal stones or peptic ulceration, polyuria, polydipsia, and mental disturbance; best remembered as bones, stones, groans, and abdominal moans.

Question 91

What is the diagnosis and give three causes?

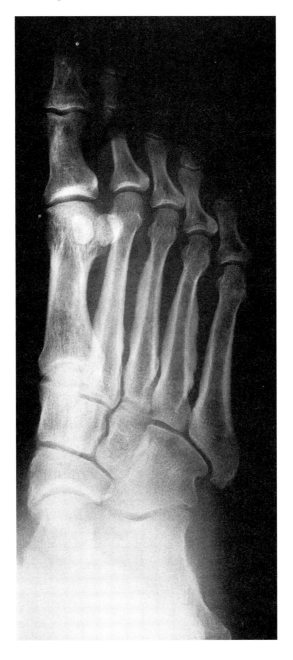

Fig. 91

Answer 91: Hypertrophic osteoarthropathy (HOA)

Findings:-There is a florid periosteal along the shafts of the 2nd to 5th metatarsals. No abnormality of the underlying bone is seen. Note the relative sparing of the metatarsal heads and bases.

Causes of HOA include:

(1) pulmonary—carcinoma of the bronchus (1 to 10%), bronchiectasis/ cystic fibrosis, empyema, metastatic deposits, and abscess;

(2) pleural—mesothelioma and pleural fibroma;

(3) abdominal—cirrhosis (especially primary biliary cirrhosis), Crohn's disease, ulcerative colitis, and biliary atresia;

(4) cardiac—cyanotic congenital heart disease;

(5) other—nasopharyngeal and oesophageal carcinoma, and infected arterial grafts.

The clinical presentation includes clubbing, joint pain, and soft tissue swelling. The commonest cause is carcinoma of the bronchus. Pleural fibroma has the highest incidence of associated HOA but is itself rare.

Radiographic changes are seen in the tibia, fibula, radius, and ulna in about 80% each; and in the proximal phalanges (60%), femur (50%), metacarpals/ metatarsals (40%), and humerus and distal phalanges (25%). Joint space narrowing and erosions are not seen in HOA.

Removal of the underlying cause can lead to resolution of symptoms within 24 hours. The radiographic changes take longer to resolve. If the primary lesion recurs, the HOA may be exacerbated.

Question 92

This 23-year-old patient suffered from a chronic condition. What abnormalities are present and what is the diagnosis?

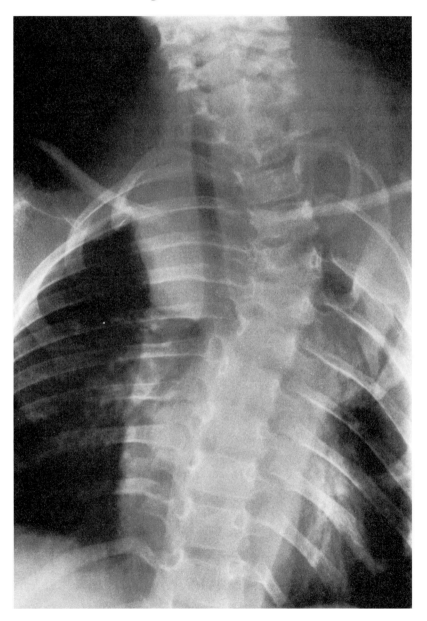

Fig. 92

Answer 92: Neurofibromatosis

Findings: There is a scoliosis concave to the right. Ribbon ribs are seen. A right posterior mediastinal mass (neurogenic tumour) extends superiorly through the thoracic inlet into the soft tissues of the neck. A left sided cervical/ chest wall mass (neurofibroma) is also present.

Neurofibromatosis (NF) is an autosomal dominant disorder. There are two types, with type 1 accounting for 90%. The gene for type 1 is located on chromosome 17 whereas that for type 2 is on chromosome 22.

Type 1 NF—diagnostic criteria (two or more of following):

- six or more cafe-au-lait spots (> 5 mm in diameter in prepubertal and >15 mm in the postpubertal);
- two or more neurofibromas;
- axillary freckling;
- one plexiform neurofibroma;
- two or more iris hamartomas (Lisch nodules);
- optic glioma;
- bone lesions, sphenoid dysplasia, or tibial pseudoarthrosis;
- one or more first degree relatives with NF-1.

Type 2 NF—diagnostic criteria (one of the following):

- bilateral acoustic neuromas;
- unilateral acoustic neuroma in association with any two of the following—meningioma, neurofibroma, schwannoma;
- unilateral acoustic neuroma with other spinal or brain tumours, of the above list, in a first degree relative.

Question 93

This 40-year-old man with chronic back pain noticed that his urine darkened when left standing. What is the diagnosis and what other radiological features may be seen?

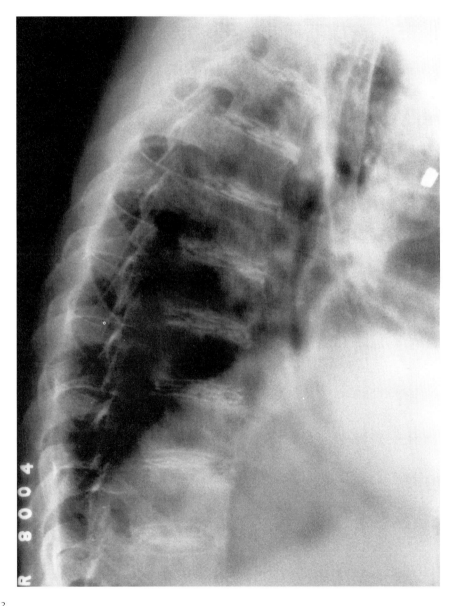

Fig. 93

Answer 93: Alkaptonuria (ochronosis)

Findings: There is intervertebral disc calcification seen at multiple levels associated with degenerative disease as evidenced by vertebral endplate sclerosis, loss of disc height, and marginal osteophytes. The vertebrae are diffusely osteopenic. Although there are many causes of intervertebral disc calcification, multiple discal involvement at such a young age is virtually pathognomonic of this condition.

Other radiological features are:

(1) chondrocalcinosis especially affecting the shoulders, hips, and knees resulting in premature degenerative arthropathy with intra-articular loose bodies;
(2) calcification of cartilage, bursas, and tendons;
(3) calcification of the aortic and mitral valves;
(4) renal calculi, nephrocalcinosis, and prostatic hypertrophy with calculi;
(5) osteoporosis.

Alkaptonuria is autosomal recessively inherited and is due to an absence of homogentisic acid oxidase resulting in a deposition of a black pigment (derivative of homogentisic acid) in the connective tissues. Premature atherosclerosis is a prominent feature. Pigment deposition also causes a bluish tinge of the ears and nasal cartilage, grey pigmentation of the sclera, and cutaneous pigmentation.

Question 94

This 26-year-old West Indian lady gave a 2-year history of increasing breathlessness and had recently developed pain in the joints of her hands. What is the diagnosis?

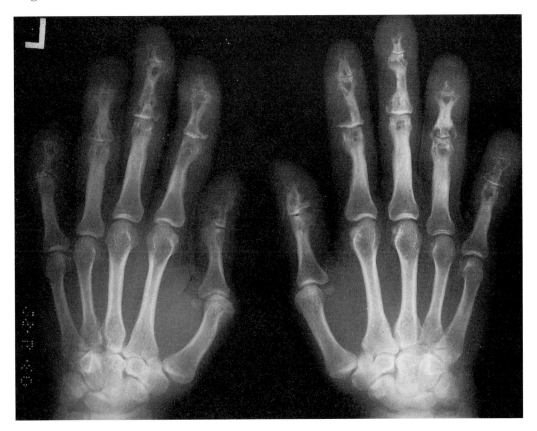

Fig. 94

Answer 94: Sarcoid osteopathy

Findings: There are multiple lytic cysts in the phalanges, with sclerotic margins, with a background lace-like trabecular pattern. The cysts are associated with bony destruction, most marked in the terminal and middle phalanges. The cysts are predominantly centrally placed in the distal ends of the phalanges. There is a dactylitis as evidenced by digital soft tissue swelling. Bone density is well preserved.

Bony involvement occurs in 5 to 10% of sarcoid patients and is usually associated with cutaneous lesions. Therefore in the absence of skin changes, radiographs are unnecessary. The hands and feet are the most common joints affected. As well as the above typical pattern, other bony changes may be seen: terminal phalangeal sclerosis, resorption of the distal phalanges, periarticular soft tissue calcification, subperiosteal bone resorption, dactylitis, and periosteal reaction. The skull and nasal bones may be involved and in the spine osteolytic lesions with loss of disc space and paraspinal masses may mimic tuberculosis. Sarcoid of the bone is an indication for systemic steroid therapy.

Question 95

This 75-year-old man with long-standing bone pain developed increasing pain in the right pelvis of recent onset. What abnormality is present and what is the diagnosis?

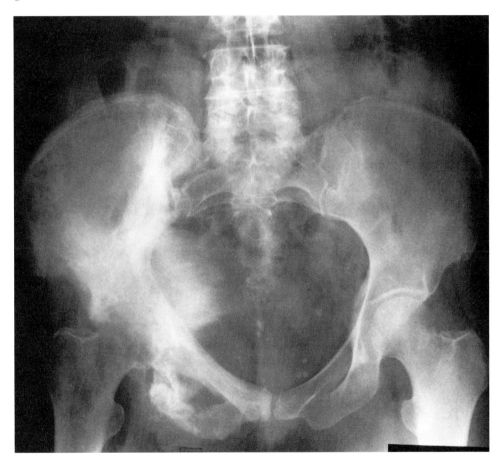

Fig. 95

Answer 95: Osteosarcoma complicating Paget's disease

Findings: There is sclerosis, expansion of the cortex, and a coarse trabecular pattern of the right hemipelvis. Thickening of the iliopectineal line is also seen. In addition, there is a destructive mass in the region of the acetabulum with associated ossification extending into the right pelvic cavity. A pathological fracture of the right inferior pubic ramus is present.

Paget's disease of the bone is a disease of the elderly and is characterized by three stages. The initial, active osteolytic phase is seen in the skull as osteoporosis circumscripta and in the long bones as a well-defined, flame-shaped advancing lucency which begins at an articular margin. The next phase is a mixed osteolytic and sclerotic stage seen in the long bones as epiphyseal and metaphyseal sclerosis with a diaphyseal lucency. The third, inactive phase is characterized by osteosclerosis with bony expansion and coarsened trabeculas. Bowing of the long bones is seen. Paget's disease most commonly involves the spine, pelvis, skull, and proximal femora. It is usually polyostotic and asymmetric.

Complications are:

(1) fractures which occur on the convexity of long bones (banana fracture);
(2) bone softening, despite increased density, resulting in bowing, basilar invagination, and protusio acetabuli;
(3) sarcomatous change (<1%)—osteosarcoma (50%), fibrosarcoma (25%), and chondrosarcoma (10%);
(4) neurological complications with cranial nerve entrapment and spinal cord compression;
(5) high output cardiac failure;
(6) degenerative joint disease.

Treatment of Paget's disease consists of analgesia, biphosphonates, and calcitonin. Disease activity may be monitored by the serum alkaline phosphatase.

Question 96

What is the differential diagnosis in this 70-year-old lady and how would you confirm it?

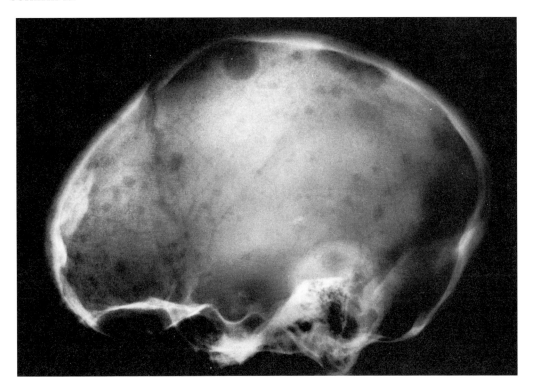

Fig. 96

Answer 96: (1) Multiple myeloma, (2) Multiple lytic metastases

Findings: There are multiple lytic lesions in the skull vault.

The diagnosis of myeloma is based on the presence of two of the following three criteria: a serum paraprotein, urinary Bence-Jones protein, and lytic bone lesions. Lytic bony metastases are most commonly from bronchus, breast, renal, and thyroid carcinoma.

Plasma cell tumours of bone are multiple (myeloma) in 94% and solitary (plasmacytoma) in 3%. Myeloma in the skeleton can exhibit a number of patterns:

(1) the commonest form (60%) is with multiple lucencies in the skull, pelvis, spine, ribs, and long bones. These are usually fairly uniform in size, unlike metastases. Vertebral body collapse is common but involvement of the pedicles is rare compared to metastases. Pathological fractures are common.

(2) generalized osteopenia without focal lesions—10 to 20%;

(3) normal—20%;

(4) multiple osteosclerotic lesions—2%;

(5) permeative bony destruction—rare.

A radionuclide bone scan is very sensitive in the detection of bony metastases but is commonly negative in myeloma because of the lack of osteoblastic activity.

Question 97

This is the left foot of a 56-year-old man with a chronic disorder. What abnormalities are present? What is the underlying cause?

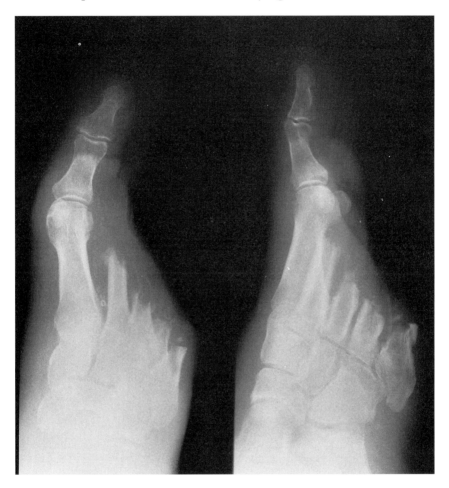

Fig. 97

Answer 97: Diabetic foot

Findings: Amputation of the 2nd to 5th toes has been performed (for gangrene). The distal aspects of the 2nd to 5th metatarsal remnants have irregular destroyed margins with a periosteal reaction, consistent with osteomyelitis. There is associated vascular calcification. These are the features of a diabetic foot.

The musculoskeletal manifestations of diabetes mellitus (DM) include:

1. Vascular calcification.
2. Osteomyelitis and septic arthritis: these processes develop when infection spreads from infected ulcers. The pressure points of the calcaneus and 1st and 5th metatarsophalangeal joints are the most common sites.
3. 'Charcot joint' (neuropathic osteoarthropathy)—the tarsometatarsal, intertarsal, and metatarsophalangeal joints are the most frequently involved.
4. Carpal tunnel syndrome—the frequency is 5 to 15% in patients with DM.
5. Osteopenia—this is particularly marked in younger patients and those requiring insulin.
6. Flexor tendon tenosynovitis.
7. Forefoot osteolysis.
8. Skeletal muscle infarction.
9. Periarthritis—patients develop a painful, stiff shoulder. The condition is up to five times more common in diabetics.
10. Gout—there is a possible association, which may be related to the high frequency of obesity in patients with hyperuricaemia.
11. Calcium pyrophosphate dihydrate deposition disease—there may be an association.

Question 98

This 72-year-old man presented with intermittent asymmetrical joint pain and swelling in the feet. Describe the abnormalities present. What is the diagnosis?

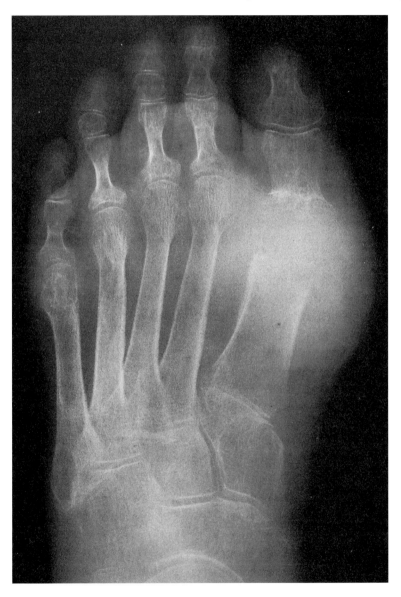

Fig. 98

Answer 98: Gout

Findings: There is marked soft-tissue swelling around the first metatarsophalangeal (MTP) joint. Well defined, 'punched-out' juxta-articular erosions are seen affecting the first proximal phalanx with more ill-defined destructive change at the first metatarsal head. Further erosions are seen at the third MTP joint. The bones are diffusely osteopenic secondary to disuse because of pain.

Gout results from the deposition of monosodium urate monohydrate crystals in the synovial membranes, articular cartilage, ligaments, and bursas resulting in cartilage destruction.

Clinically there are three stages. An initial asymptomatic hyperuricaemic phase—20% of this group will develop renal calculi or joint disease. The next stage is that of acute gouty arthritis. This is usually a mono- or oligoarticular process, but may be polyarticular. The third stage is chronic tophaceous gout. There is a predilection for the lower limb. The first metatarsophalangeal joint is the most commonly affected (70%). Gouty tophi occur at the ears, tendons, and bursas. The initial radiological sign is periarticular swelling from the joint effusion and/or tophi. Subsequently, erosive disease develops. Erosions at an involved joint are seen to have over-hanging margins and some surrounding sclerosis (unlike rheumatoid arthritis). The distribution of the affected joints, well preserved joint space (due to the relatively late destruction of the articular cartilage), and the absence of periarticular osteopenia also help to differentiate gout from rheumatoid.

Question 99

This 44-year-old Asian lady presented with bone pain, particularly affecting the hips, and non-specific muscle weakness. What abnormalities are shown and what is the underlying diagnosis?

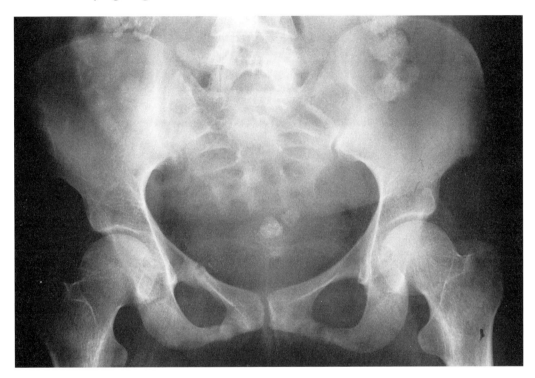

Fig. 99

Answer 99: Osteomalacia

Findings: Looser's zones are present in both inferior pubic rami and the right superior pubic ramus.

Osteomalacia results from an abnormality of vitamin D metabolism. Excess, uncalcified osteoid accumulates and the bones become soft. The bone softening may lead to: long bone bowing, pelvic and thoracic cage deformity, and biconcave vertebral bodies or fractures. Looser's zones are 2 to 3 mm thick radiolucencies representing osteoid formed within stress-induced infractions. They are usually bilateral, symmetrical, and perpendicular to the bony cortex: common sites are the medial femoral neck, lateral border of the scapula, pubic rami, and ribs.

The clinical features on presentation are often non-specific but bone pain and tenderness with muscular weakness may be present. Serum examination shows a low/ normal calcium, a low phosphate, and an elevated alkaline phosphatase.

Worldwide the commonest cause of osteomalacia is dietary vitamin D deficiency. Malabsorption is a common cause in the United Kingdom, for example coeliac disease, pancreatic insufficiency, biliary disease, and gastric surgery. Chronic renal failure leads to osteomalacia by decreased conversion of 25-hydroxycholecalciferol (25(OH)D) to 1,25-dihydroxycholecalciferol. Other causes are liver disease and anticonvulsant therapy. Inherited causes include X-linked vitamin D resistant rickets.

Question 100

This 1-year-old presented with a 2-week history of refusing to weight bear. What is the diagnosis?

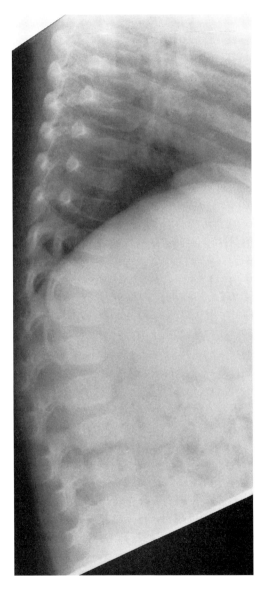

Fig. 100

Answer 100: Discitis at L3/4

Findings: There is loss of the L3/4 disc space associated with destruction of the inferior end-plate of L3 and the superior endplate of L4.

Infective spondylitis usually affects males and is most common in the 40 to 50 year-old age group. Lumbar (especially L3–4 and L4–5) involvement is most common, followed by thoracic disease. In adults, infection usually begins as an anterosuperior, or anteroinferior sub-chondral focus, seen as a lytic lesion. This may then spread to involve (sequentially) the adjacent disc space (with destruction of the end plates and loss of disc space), adjacent vertebral body, subligamentous paravertebral space, and then the paraspinal soft tissues. The source of infection may be haematogenous (this may follow urogenital or gastrointestinal tract infection), contiguous suppurative focus, and traumatic or iatrogenic direct inoculation. *Staphylococcus aureus* is the most common organism in Caucasians and tuberculosis in Asians. Direct aspiration is usually required to obtain proof of the causative organism.

A radionuclide bone scan is very sensitive at localizing bony abnormalities but is non-specific as regards aetiology. CT is more sensitive than plain films in demonstrating the lytic bone change and soft tissue mass. MR (Fig. 100a) is the most appropriate investigation as it is extremely sensitive in detecting bony and discal pathology (before abnormalities are seen on the plain film) as well as demonstrating spinal canal involvement.

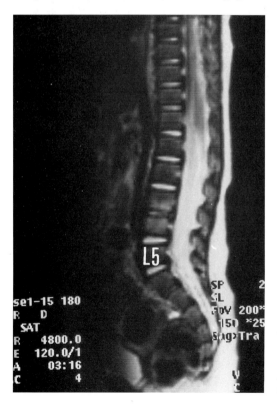

Fig. 100a Sagittal T2 weighted thoracolumbar spine (L5 labelled). There is a discitis at the L3/4 level with loss of disc space and normal signal (compare to the other intervertebral discs). Abnormal high signal is present in the adjacent vertebral bodies indicative of marrow oedema.

Question 101

What is the diagnosis?

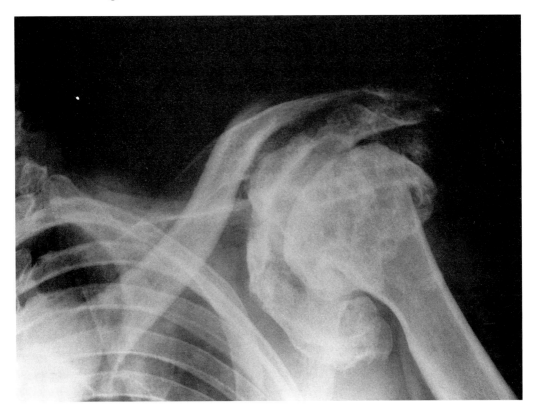

Fig. 101

Answer 101: Neuropathic (Charcot) joint

Findings: The radiological features of a neuropathic joint are the '5 Ds': Dense (heterotropic new bone beneath the site of the articular cartilage), Destruction (of the articular cortex), Deformity, Debris (loose bodies within the joint), and Dislocation.

Conditions which may give rise to a neuropathic joint include:

(1)   congenital (spina bifida and indifference to pain);
(2)   acquired:

     (a)   neural axis lesion—trauma, tumour, syphilis (20% of patients with tabes dorsalis, especially joints of lower limbs), and syringomyelia (33% of patients, especially shoulder joint);

     (b)   peripheral neuropathy—diabetes mellitus (most common, especially affecting hands and feet), leprosy, and trauma.

Question 102

This 68-year-old lady complained of generalized aches and pains. What is the diagnosis?

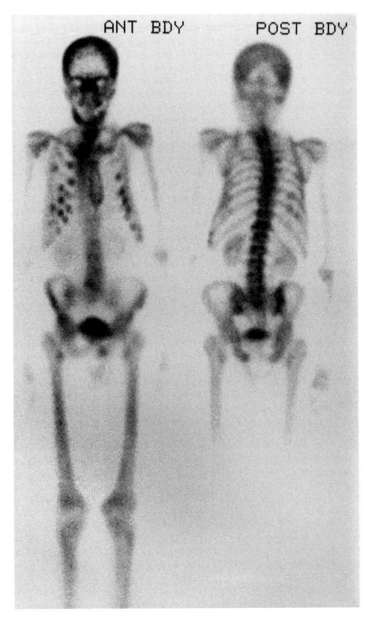

Fig. 102

Answer 102: 'Superscan' due to osteomalacia

Findings: There is increased tracer uptake throughout the skeleton with decreased renal uptake. Looser's zones are seen in the medial aspects of both femoral necks and left inferior pubic ramus. There is increased tracer uptake at the costochondral junctions (rickety rosary), the distribution of which is not random, as seen in metastatic disease and is too extensive to suggest trauma. A scoliosis is present.

A superscan occurs in the presence of a diffuse bone pathology resulting in an increased bone to soft tissue radionuclide uptake ratio. The commonest cause of a superscan is widespread metastatic disease (Fig. 102a). In metastatic disease, the increased uptake may be uniform but there is commonly inhomogeneity of the ribs or skull. The most common primary neoplasms are: breast, lung, and prostate. Other causes of a superscan include:

- renal osteodystrophy;
- hyperparathyroidism (focal uptake at brown tumours);
- hyperthyroidism;
- myelofibrosis and myelosclerosis;
- mastocytosis;
- Paget's disease (rarely).

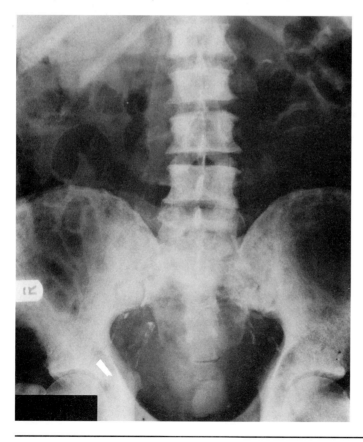

Fig. 102a   Radiograph of the pelvis and lumbosacral spine of a 78-year-old man showing diffusely dense bones due to metastatic carcinoma of prostate.

Question 103

This 32-year-old intravenous drug abuser (IVDA) presented with a painful right hip. What is the most likely diagnosis?

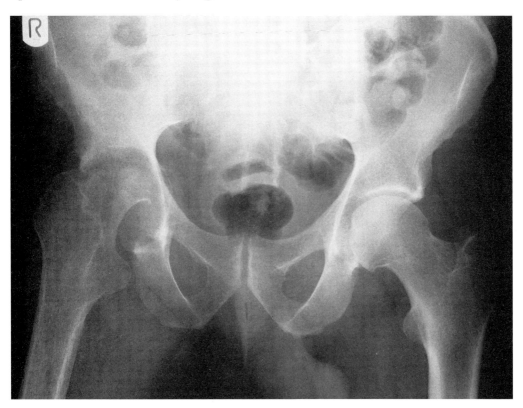

Fig. 103

Answer 103: Septic arthritis of the right hip

Findings: There is extensive destruction of the right femoral head and the acetabulum with loss of normal joint space. The femur is superiorly subluxed. The coronal T1 weighted MRI (Fig. 103a) shows low signal return from the right femoral head (black arrow) and acetabulum with synovial thickening and a joint effusion (arrowheads). There is an associated protusio acetabuli.

Septic arthritis is most commonly seen in children. The routes of contamination of joints are:

(1)   haematogenous (direct synovial infection by septic emboli);
(2)   spread from adjacent bone (intra-articular extension from adjacent osteomyelitis);
(3)   direct inoculation, for example postoperatively, aspiration, or penetrating injury (needles in IVDAs).

Initially, synovial thickening and effusion distend the joint with displacement of the periarticular fat planes. The joint effusion may easily be detected on ultrasound and diagnostic aspiration performed. The next stage is cartilage destruction with accompanying loss of joint space. This is followed by osseous erosion on both sides of the joint with separation of bone ends, subluxation, and dislocation in severe cases. During recovery, fibrous or bony ankylosis may result. MR is very sensitive in the detection of cartilaginous and periarticular bone marrow changes. CT optimally demonstrates bony involvement before they become evident on plain film. Triple phase dynamic bone scans are abnormal within hours to days of the onset of infection but are not specific. Labelled white cell scans are useful in the evaluation of joint prostheses, differentiating infection from loosening.

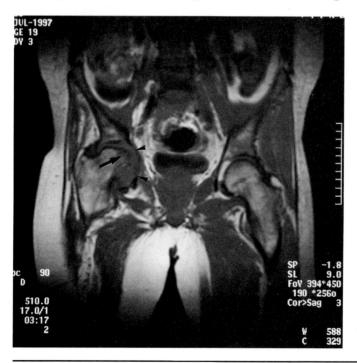

Fig. 103a   Coronal T1 weighted MRI showing a septic arthritis of the right hip.

Question 104

These sagittal T1 weighted images are of a 55-year-old lady with an acute exacerbation of chronic low back pain. The L5 and S1 vertebral bodies are indicated. What is the diagnosis?

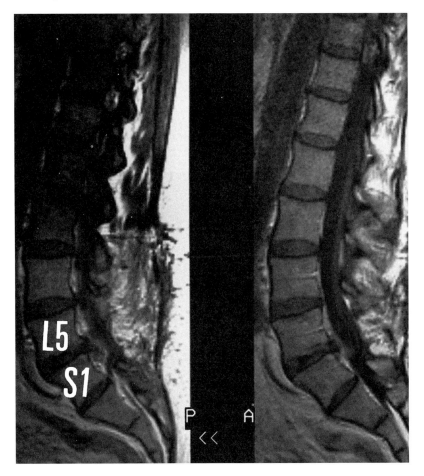

Fig. 104

Answer 104: L5-S1 disc prolapse

Findings: The L5-S1 disc shows signal change and loss of height, in keeping with degeneration. At the L5-S1 level there is a large disc prolapse posteriorly into the spinal canal (arrows, Fig. 104a).

Disc herniation is defined as a focal protrusion of discal material (nucleus pulposus) beyond the margins of adjacent vertebral endplates and is secondary to a tear of the annulus fibrosus. A disc herniation may impinge upon the roots within the spinal canal or in their exiting neural foramina resulting in radicular signs.

MR is the imaging modality of choice for demonstrating disc bulges and herniations. MRI shows discal herniation into the spinal canal or neural exit foramina better than CT or myelography. It is also able to distinguish postoperative scarring from disc herniation with a high degree of accuracy. Disc herniation is common; at least one is found in 33% of asymptomatic patients aged over 60 years. Of disc herniations, 90% are at L4-5 or L5-S1, and 95% are inside the spinal canal (the rest are predominantly foraminal or extraforaminal).

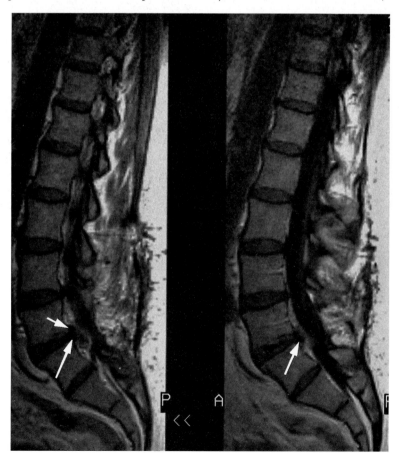

Fig. 104a Sagittal T1 weighted image of the lumbar spine showing disc prolapse at the L5-S1 level.

Question 105

This coronal T1 weighted MR image is of a 34-year-old man who presented with bilateral hip pain. What is the diagnosis? What causes are there?

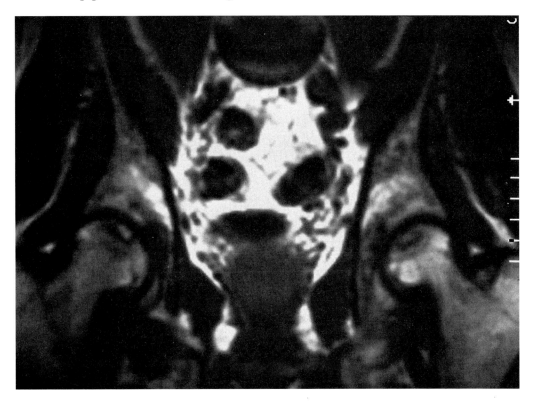

Fig. 105

Answer 105: Bilateral avascular necrosis (AVN) of the hips

Findings: There are well-defined serpiginous bands of low signal on the superomedial aspect of the femoral heads (necrotic bone marrow) with a central bright area. The appearance has been likened to a tennis ball.

There are a wide range of underlying causes of AVN. These include:

- inflammatory—rheumatoid arthritis, SLE, scleroderma, infection (following a pyogenic arthritis), and acute pancreatitis;
- toxic—steroids, alcohol;
- metabolic—diabetes mellitus, Cushing's syndrome, and pregnancy;
- traumatic—fractures (especially femoral neck, scaphoid, and talus);
- idiopathic—Perthes' disease (children 5 to 8 years old);
- haemopoietic disorders—sickle cell disease, polycythaemia rubra vera, Gaucher's disease, and haemophilia.
- thromboembolic—Caisson disease, radiotherapy, and fat embolism.

The investigation of choice for confirming the diagnosis is MR which has a 90 to 100% sensitivity and diagnosis is possible before changes become apparent on plain films (Fig. 105a). Early diagnosis allows prompt intervention when the condition is still reversible.

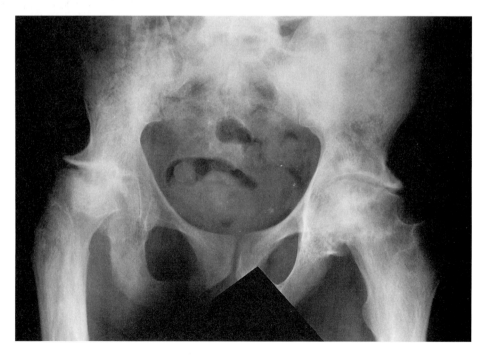

Fig. 105a   Bilateral avascular necrosis of the hips. There is sclerosis and irregularity of the femoral heads with flattening and secondary degenerative changes. The bones are diffusely dense due to sickle cell disease.

Question 106

This 36-year-old gave a long history of pain in the joints of his hands and a skin rash. What is the diagnosis?

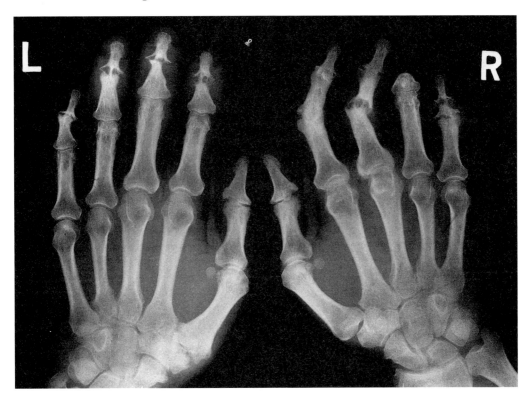

Fig. 106

Answer 106: Psoriatic arthropathy

Findings: There is an asymmetrical erosive arthropathy affecting the distal interphalangeal (DIP) joints of both hands. At the proximal interphalangeal (PIP) joints of the right 2nd and 3rd digits the erosive changes have produced a 'cup and pencil' deformity. There is telescoping of the right 4th digit. There is soft tissue swelling of the fingers. Bone density is well preserved.

Arthropathy occurs in 5% of psoriatics and may precede skin changes. The erosions in psoriatic arthropathy are subarticular, compared to periarticular in rheumatoid arthritis, and are associated with marked adjacent new bone formation. At distal phalangeal bases, a bat's wing appearance results. It is typically asymmetrical and may be associated with periosteal new bone formation. Cartilage loss and ankylosis of the joints may occur.

Five patterns of psoriatic arthropathy are recognized:

(1)   monoarthritis or asymmetrical oligoarthritis (70%);
(2)   rheumatoid arthritis pattern (15%);
(3)   polyarthritis mainly affecting the DIP joints (5%);
(4)   spondyloarthritis mimicking ankylosing spondylitis;
(5)   arthritis mutilans.

Question 107

This 78-year-old man presented with weight loss. What is the diagnosis?

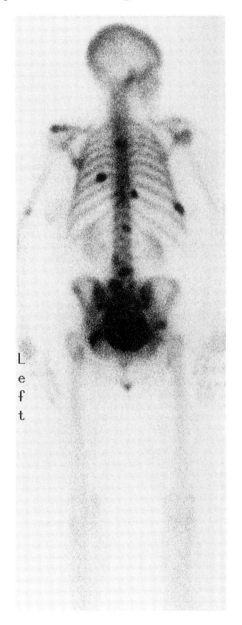

Fig. 107

Answer 107: Metastatic disease (from carcinoma of the lung)

Findings: Multiple, randomly scattered foci of increased tracer uptake are present.

A malignant bone lesion in an adult is more likely to be metastatic than primary. Metastases have a predilection for the axial skeleton. When there is a known primary lesion, it is breast in 35%, prostate in 30%, lung in 10%, kidney in 5%, thyroid in 2%, and others in 18%. If the primary tumour is unknown, it will later be shown to be prostate in 25%, lymphoma in 15%, breast in 10%, lung in 10%, and other/ not identified in 40%.

If a solitary 'hot spot' is found on a bone scan of a patient with no known malignancy, there is a 5% chance that it represents a metastatic deposit. If a solitary lesion is seen in a patient with a known malignancy, there is a 50% chance that it represents a metastasis. Five percent of metastatic bony deposits show no abnormality on a bone scan.

Question 108

This 38-year-old lady was referred for ultrasound with a suspected deep vein thrombosis. This ultrasound image is taken longitudinally behind the knee. Cephalad is to the left of the image and the caudad is to the right. What has been measured and what is the diagnosis?

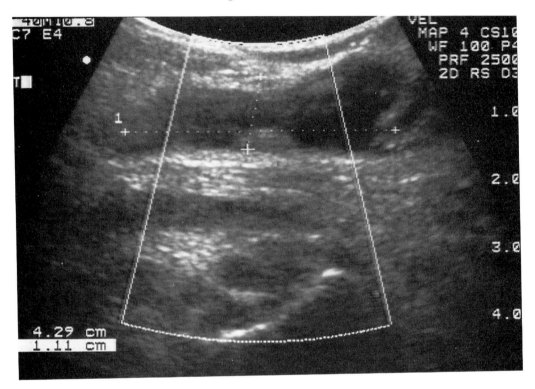

Fig. 108

Answer 108: Baker's cyst (ruptured)

Findings: A Baker's cyst has been measured. To the right of the cyst there is some free fluid (black streaks) in the muscles of the calf confirming rupture of the cyst. Anterior to the cyst (below the cyst on this image) is a tubular structure which is the patent popliteal vein. Note the colour doppler box for assessing vessel patency. Anterior to the vein, the posterior aspect of the tibia is seen.

A Baker's cyst is a collection of synovial fluid within a bursa (usually the gastrocnemio-semimembranous bursa at the posteromedial aspect of the knee). The bursa communicates with the knee joint and is formed secondary to raised intra-articular pressure associated with a knee effusion, usually due to an arthritic process. Rupture of the bursa mimics a deep venous thrombosis and it is important to exclude it to avoid inappropriate anticoagulation. Following rupture of the cyst, there is an increased risk of venous thrombosis due to impeded venous return and immobility.

Question 109

This 16-year-old girl was under investigation for short stature and precocious puberty. What abnormalities are present and what is the diagnosis?

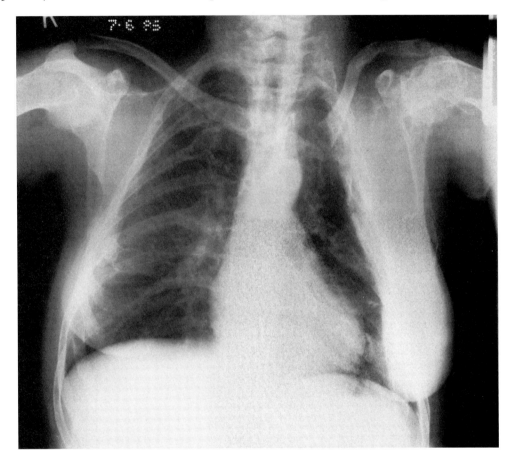

Fig. 109

Answer 109: Polyostotic fibrous dysplasia (McCune–Albright's disease)

Findings: There are well-defined, expanded lesions of multiple ribs with a 'ground-glass' appearance. The lesions exhibit endosteal scalloping (thinned cortex from within). A modelling deformity (thoracic cage deformity) is seen due to bone softening. The same features are also present in the hands (Fig. 109a).

Fibrous dysplasia is a benign mesenchymal disorder of bone. It is commonest in the first and second decades and progresses until growth ceases. It is usually monostotic (70 to 80%) but in the polyostotic variant may be associated with precocious puberty and cafe-au-lait spots (McCune—Albright's disease). Other endocrinopathies, for example hyperthyroidism, hyperparathyroidism, and hypophosphataemic rickets, may occur in the polyostotic variant. The pelvis and femur are the commonest bones affected in the polyostotic form and the ribs, femur, and tibia in the monostotic type. Complications include fracture and, rarely, malignant change.

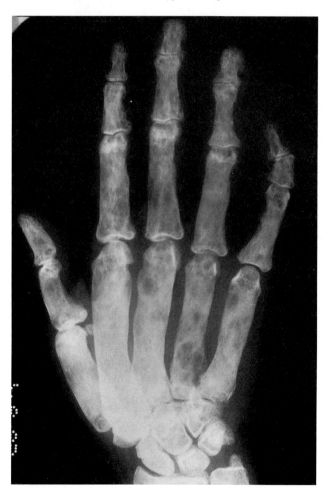

Fig. 109a Polyostotic fibrous dysplasia of the hand.

Question 110

Which disease is most likely to be the cause of this appearance?

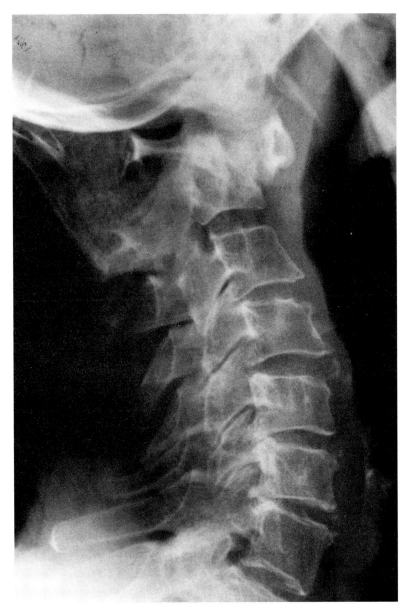

Fig. 110

Answer 110: *Rheumatoid arthritis*

Findings: There is erosion of the odontoid peg with subluxation of the atlantoaxial joint. There are secondary degenerative changes as shown by narrowing of the disc spaces at several levels with osteophyte formation. In contrast, osteoarthritis of the cervical spine predominantly affects the C5/6 and C6/7 levels. There is calcification of the nuchal membrane.

A separation in the atlantoaxial joint space of greater than 3 mm, in adults, is abnormal. It occurs in about 6% of rheumatoid patients. In rheumatoid arthritis, atlantoaxial subluxation occurs because of weakening and laxity of the transverse ligament caused by pannus from the synovial bursa adjacent to the odontoid peg. The pannus may erode the peg. Spinal cord compression may ensue. In less florid cases, flexion views of the cervical spine may produce the subluxation and these should be performed prior to general anaesthesia. Rheumatoid cervical spondylitis is also characterized by multiple disc space narrowing and subluxation due to involvement of the joints of Luschka (at the lateral margins of the cervical vertebral bodies) and ligamentous weakening.

Other causes of atlantoaxial subluxation are:

(1) connective tissue diseases—ankylosing spondylitis, Reiter's syndrome, psoriatic arthropathy, SLE, and juvenile chronic arthritis;
(2) trauma (very rare without odontoid fracture);
(3) infection—retropharyngeal abscess in children;
(4) congenital—Down's syndrome, Morquio's syndrome.

Bibliography

Armstrong, P., Wilson, A.G., Dee, P., and Hansell, D.M. (1995). *Imaging of diseases of the chest*, (2nd edn). Mosby, St. Louis.

Dahnert, W. (1996). *Radiology review manual*, (3rd edn). Williams and Wilkins Baltimore.

Grainger, R.G. and Allison, D.J. (1997). *Diagnostic radiology: a textbook of medical imaging*, (3rd edn). Churchill Livingstone Edinburgh.

Resnick, D. (1989). *Bone and joint imaging*. Saunders Philadelphia.

Sutton, D. (1993). A *textbook of radiology and imaging*, (5th edn). Churchill Livingstone, Edinburgh.

Index (by subject)

question numbers are in bold